FLYING CLOTHING
The story of its development

D1342

D1342

FLYING CLOTHING

The story of its development

Louise Greer
and Anthony Harold

Illustrations by Anthony Harold

Airlife
England

Airlife Publishing Ltd.

7, St John's Hill, Shrewsbury, England

Printed in England by Livesey Ltd., Shrewsbury

Contents

Foreword

by MARSHAL OF THE ROYAL AIR FORCE,
SIR DERMOT BOYLE,
GCB KCVO KBE AFC

This is more than a record of the development of flying clothing. It touches on the evolution of manned flight and is of lively interest for this alone. It is also a serious well-researched story of how and why aircrew have come to clothe and equip themselves as they have over the years.

    This book fills a gap in aviation history and in doing so brings to light many amusing and long-forgotten incidents. It is therefore of interest to both the flying enthusiast and those who wish to know all there is to know about flying clothing.

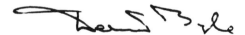

Introduction

When one thinks of aviation one automatically thinks of the rapid advances in the development of airframes and aero engines and of the numerous types of aircraft that have evolved over the last seventy years. Rarely does one think of the human operator; maybe because man has changed so little. However, man was not born to fly. His natural habitat is not 35,000 ft above the earth. At altitude the atmosphere is an environment hostile to man, and an aircraft is not always a placid playfellow. Man's body is very adaptable but it does have its physiological limitations and these are at no time more apparent than when it is being hurtled heavenwards.

The efficiency of the man-machine combination depends entirely upon that of each individual part. Thus every effort must be made to ensure that the pilot is as comfortable as possible and that his operational efficiency is maintained at the maximum level. A pilot's concentration must not be impaired by any discomfort. The hostile environment must therefore be modified to meet the needs of the aviator.

Flying clothing mitigates conditions of excess heat or cold, of lack of oxygen, of lack of pressure, of violent acceleration or deceleration, of deafening noise or blinding glare. It creates an artificial environment in an attempt to prevent man's limitations from inhibiting his aircraft's performance. Flying clothing, provided in order to counteract the stresses imposed upon a pilot in flight, includes emergency equipment such as parachutes, life-jackets, immersion suits, and other equipment worn on or restricting the body.

Flying clothing is essentially functional, and its development closely related to that of the aircraft. Rapid strides have been made in both spheres. An aviator of the first decade of this century would not only find it difficult to relate to the supersonic military aircraft hurtling through the stratosphere but would also find it well-nigh impossible to identify himself with the Martian-like figure at the controls.

In this book we have concentrated mainly on the development of flying clothing in Britain, both standard and experimental, but with special emphasis on the military aspect, since military requirements have, on the whole, been more demanding and military research more significant. We do look at innovations by other nations, and, when operating in close proximity to them such as during the war years, we observe their standard flying kit.

In spite of the lack of much of the original material, we hope that this book will shed some light on the human factor in the field of flight and that it will fill a gap in the information available on this interesting subject.

1979

Louise Greer
A. C. Harold

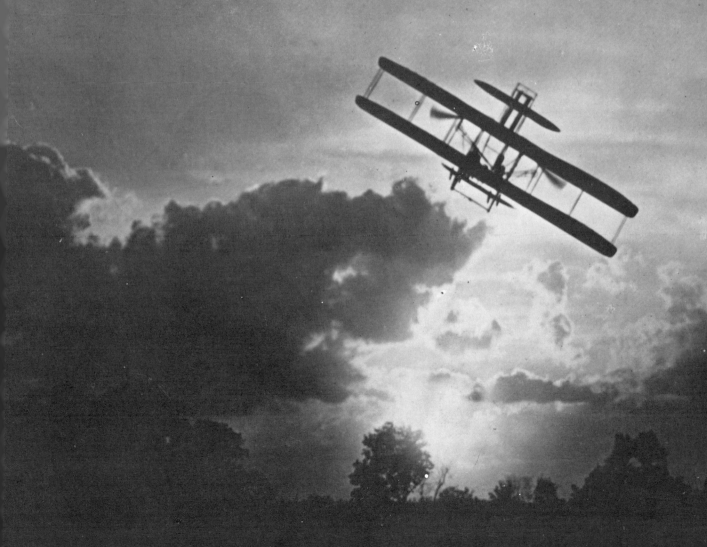

CHAPTER 1
A DREAM COMES TRUE

For centuries birds have tantalised man. Effortless flight–compared with the inelegant earthbound walk. The dreams of flight are as old as mankind itself, but it was not until 1783 that man discovered a successful means of taking to the air. In that year the Montgolfier brothers, owners of a paper mill near Annonay in France, designed an enormous paper and linen balloon which, when inflated with hot air given off from burning straw, reached an estimated height of 6,000ft. Many spectators were present to watch this triumph, and the news spread rapidly through Europe. Only two months later Professor Charles of the Académie Française, who was familiar with Henry Cavendish's work on hydrogen, decided to obtain lift by filling a balloon with this gas rather than with hot air; this achieved a similar success. Although neither the Montgolfière nor Charlière balloon was able to carry any passengers it was not long before cargoes were carried skywards.

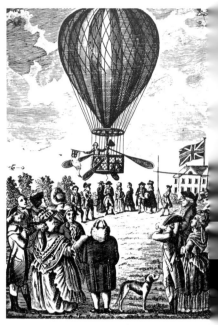

Lunardi's ascent from Moorfields, 1784
The first manned balloon ascent in England

The first aerial passengers were a sheep, a duck and a cockerel, which ascended in a beautiful green and gold Montgolfière hot-air balloon, all occupants fortunately landing safely. The duck and cockerel were of course impeccably dressed for flying, and the sheep was warmly dressed in wool, an example followed by many later aviators. This flight encouraged the director of the French Royal Museum, Pilâtre de Rozier, and his friend the Marquis d'Arlandes to attempt to become the first men to ascend in a balloon; they drifted for six miles over Paris in a Montgolfière in October 1783. When Professor Charles publicly announced he was planning an ascent from the Tuileries on 1 December 1783, two-thirds of Paris came to watch this new and amazing spectacle. After a brief flight with a Monsieur Robert, Professor Charles ascended alone. His account of the experience is graphic:

> I passed in ten minutes from the temperature of spring to that of winter; the cold was keen and dry, but not insupportable. I examined all my sensations calmly; I could hear myself live, so to speak, and I am certain that at first I experienced nothing disagreeable in this sudden passage from one temperature to another.
>
> When the barometer ceased to fall I noted very exactly eighteen inches ten lines. From this I deduce a height of 1,524 toises (3,100 yds). In a few minutes more my fingers were benumbed by the cold, so that I could not hold my pen. I was now stationary, or rather moved only in a horizontal direction.
>
> I raised myself in the middle of the car, and abandoned myself to the spectacle before me. At my departure from the meadow the sun had sunk to the people of the valleys; soon he shone for me alone, and came again to pour his rays upon the balloon and the car. I was the only creature in the horizon in sunshine–all the rest of nature was in shade. 'Ere long, however, the sun disappeared, and thus I had the pleasure of seeing him set twice in the same day. I contemplated for some moments the mists and vapours that rose from the valley and the rivers. The clouds seemed to come forth from the earth, and to accumulate the one upon the other. Their colour was a monotonous grey–a natural effect, for there was no light save that of the moon.
>
> I observed that I had tacked round twice, and I felt currents which called me to my senses. I found with surprise the effect of the wind, and saw the cloth of my flag extended horizontally.
>
> In the midst of the inexpressible pleasure of this state of ecstatic contemplation, I was recalled to myself by a most extraordinary pain which I felt in the interior of the ears and in the maxillary glands. This I attributed to the dilation of the air contained in the cellular tissue of the organ as much as to the cold outside. I was in my waistcoat, with my head uncovered. I immediately covered my head with a bonnet of wool which was at my feet, but the pain only disappeared with my descent to the ground.
>
> It was now seven or eight minutes since I had arrived at this elevation, and I now commenced to descend. I remembered the promise I had made to the Duke of Chartres, to return in half an hour.

Poor Professor Charles was the first of many aviators who in flight were to suffer the effects of extreme cold, learning the hard way that a waistcoat and woollen bonnet were inadequate protection against the severe cold encountered at altitude, for the temperature falls by approximately 2°C for every 1,000ft.

One of the most colourful ballooning figures of the eighteenth century was Vincent Lunardi, a dashing young Italian diplomat based in London who in 1784 made the first aerial ascent in England. He drifted in a Charlière or hydrogen balloon from the Artillery Ground at Moorfields to South Mimms in Buckinghamshire, accompanied by a dog, a cat and a pigeon. Lunardi always ascended in the dress of the Honourable Artillery Company, of which he was a member; this consisted of bright red and blue tunic and trousers, plus a tricorne hat trimmed with red velvet and gold lace. Like Charles he, too, felt the cold, but Lunardi had what became a commonplace solution to the problem.

> When the thermometer had fallen from 68° to 61° I perceived a great difference in the temperature of the air. I became very cold, and found it necessary to take a few glasses of wine. I likewise ate the leg of a chicken, but my bread and other provisions had been rendered useless, by being mixed with sand, which I carried as ballast.
> I moved to different parts of the gallery, I adjusted the furniture, and apparatus. I uncorked my bottle, ate, drank and wrote, just as in my study.

Lunardi supported the popular theory that oars were necessary for the balloon to move horizontally through the air. Thus he heartily 'rowed' his way along, not realising that the paddles had no effect other than keeping him warm and alert. Lunardi travelled round England making famous ascents from Liverpool to Edinburgh, watched by clamouring mobs and wide-eyed swooning women. When he flew across the Firth of Forth he is said to have worn a special life-saving cork jacket provided by a Dr Rae. This is the first recorded instance of the wearing of a life jacket in flight.

His fame soon spread, and people travelled many miles, paying vast sums of money to see this stunning Italian rise from the earth in his brightly coloured balloon. Poems were dedicated to him and bonnets and skirts named after him. When ballooning started in England, the Church claimed that the aeronauts would be damned for rising heavenwards before their appointed time, and on several occasions when Lunardi appeared out of the skies calling over his loud-hailer for assistance, villagers fled in terror, believing him to be the Angel Gabriel.

But by 1785 ballooning was an accepted, if eccentric, sport known to all by the famous Channel crossing of J. P. Blanchard and his financial backer, Dr John Jeffries of Boston, which was later proclaimed the greatest feat of the century. They set off on their perilous voyage on a cold January day. Leaving the coast of Dover behind them they began to lose height rapidly and before long were forced to jettison all their sand ballast. For a large part of the journey they were just skimming the waves and, to avoid ditching in the Channel, they threw overboard their food, the oars, the basket lining and any other disposable equipment they could find. Dr Jeffries related:

> Nothing seemed to help, so we began to strip ourselves. Blanchard first tossed away his extra coat and surtout; and I then discarded my only coat. Blanchard next sacrificed his light coat and trousers, and by this time I was so concerned and, being a physician, I suggested that we gag ourselves and vomit up what food we had already eaten, but this was not necessary. We put on and adjusted our cork jackets and prepared for a plunge into the sea.

But luck was with them, the balloon rose and they landed safely near Calais, to a joyous welcome from the local inhabitants and an award of 12,000 francs from Louis XVI. Sir Richard Crosbie, who in January 1785 made the first balloon ascent in Ireland, was clothed rather more exotically, notably a long coat of oiled silk lined with fur, a waistcoat and breeches of quilted satin, morocco boots and a Montero leopard-skin cap.

The French Revolution was just around the corner, heralding a series of European wars and revolutions. The military could not ignore the recent aerial innovations, and as countries became embroiled in armed conflict they had to decide whether or not to adopt the balloon for military purposes. France set an example as early as 1794 when the **Public Safety Committee** of the new Republic formed an airborne unit using balloons for observation. There is no mention of the balloonists wearing other than the normal

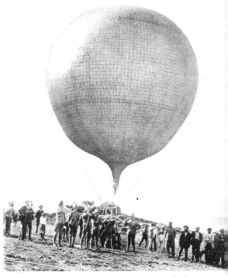

Royal Engineers about to ascend in an observation balloon at Ladysmith during the Boer War.

eighteenth-century dress. There was a hydrogen-balloon corps in the Union Army in the American Civil War of 1861–5 under Thaddeus Lowe, but the tethered balloon tended to rock fiercely in even moderate winds, making the observer airsick and unable to monitor any activities below. Balloons were used for observation in the Siege of Paris in 1870; they also carried 164 people, 381 carrier pigeons, five dogs and three million letters out of Paris over a four-month period. The British adopted aerial reconnaissance during the Boer War in South Africa, but because it was unnecessary to attain great heights for observation the officers were not unduly affected by the cold and usually ascended in their everyday working uniforms.

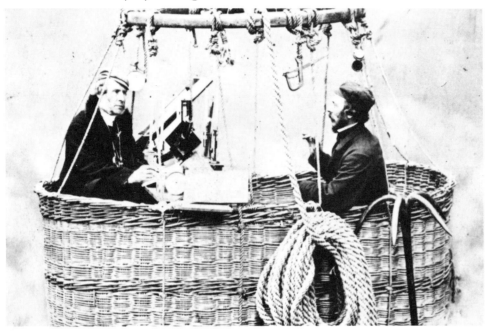

Coxwell and Glaisher posing in their balloo basket 1862.

Until the beginning of the nineteenth century balloons had not been reaching heights of more than 12,000 ft. The main problem the aeronauts encountered was that of cold, which they found could be overcome partly by the addition of extra layers of clothing. Because balloons move with the airstream the cold is not intensified by any biting wind; but temperature falls with altitude and by 10,000 ft one could expect to have to withstand minus 5°C.

When balloons started to reach heights of more than 14,000 ft aviators experienced seemingly inexplicable sensations of dizziness and faintness. These symptoms had appeared earlier in the eighteenth century when mountains such as Mont Blanc (15,781 ft) were climbed. In 1852 one foolhardy balloonist, Mr Charles Green rose, with three companions, to 19,200 ft to make meteorological observations, withstanding a temperature well below freezing point. Ten years later the British Association sponsored the ascent of Henry Coxwell, an experienced aeronaut, and James Glaisher a meteorologist by profession. They rose from Wolverhampton in their balloon the *Mammoth* to an estimated 30,000 ft. Although these early high-altitude ascents were conducted by scientists, interest lay simply in testing the characteristics of the air at those heights rather than in the effects of rarefied air on the human body. The *Mammoth* did not carry any oxygen equipment. Glaisher later explained:

Mr Green and companions 1852.

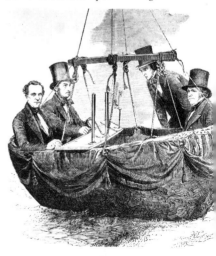

> I laid my arm upon the table, possessed of its full vigour, but on being desirous of using it I found it powerless ... Then I tried to shake myself, and succeeded, but I seemed to have no limbs ... I dimly saw Mr Coxwell, and endeavoured to speak, but could not. In an instant, intense darkness overcame me ... I thought I had been seized with asphyxia, and believed I should experience nothing more as death would come unless we speedily descended; other thoughts were entering my mind, when I suddenly became unconscious, as on going to sleep.

By some miracle Glaisher and Coxwell lived to tell the tale. But in 1875 three French-men, Ms Sivel, Gaston Tissandier and Croce-Spinelli, ascended from Paris in their balloon the *Zenith* to over 28,000 ft. Only Tissandier returned to earth alive. The flight of Tissandier and his two ill-fated companions was significant because it was one of the first scientific experiments to determine the effects of altitude on man's metabolism. Tissandier's description is very similar to Glaisher's, written thirteen years before:

> I now come to the fateful moments when we were overcome by the terrific effect of reduced pressure. At 24,000 ft the condition of torpor that overcomes me is extra-ordinary. The body and mind weaken little by little, gradually, unconsciously, without one's knowledge one does not suffer at all; on the contrary. One experiences inner joy, as if it were an effect of the inundating flood of light . . . one no longer thinks of the perilous situation or of the danger; one rises and is happy to rise . . . I soon felt myself so weak that I could not turn my head to look at my companions . . . I wished to call out that we were at 26,000 ft, but my tongue was paralysed. Suddenly I closed my eyes and fell inert, entirely losing consciousness.

This was the first time that supplies of oxygen had been carried aloft in a balloon, but unfortunately Tissandier and his companions failed to realise their need for it until they were all too weak even to reach for the oxygen tubes. When their balloon returned to earth it was discovered that the supplies of oxygen were virtually untouched.

The condition from which these balloonists had been suffering is known as hypoxia or altitude-sickness, a problem that has been encountered throughout the history of flight. Hypoxia is a term used to denote a deficiency of oxygen in the bloodstream. With increasing altitude the atmospheric pressure decreases – at sea-level it is 760 mm of mercury, whereas at 19,000 ft, for example, it is only 364 mm. Hypoxia is not due to a decreased percentage of oxygen in the air but to a decreased partial pressure of oxygen in the lungs. The pressure in the lungs is too low to force the gas into solution in the blood. As the

Hedges Butler, founder of the Royal Aero Club, preparing for a balloon ascent from Wandsworth 1906.

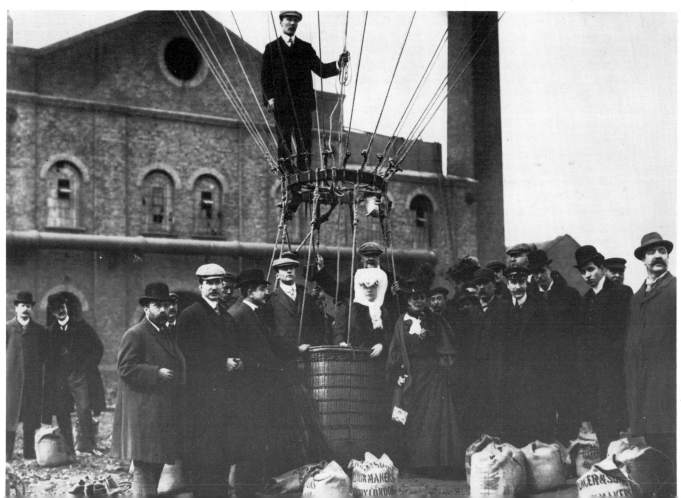

partial pressure of oxygen falls with altitude so less oxygen is diffused into the blood-stream and the body ceases to function properly. The symptoms of hypoxia vary from one person to another, depending on physical fitness, on the altitude reached and on the length of time spent there. Some of these symptoms are dizziness, lack of breath, head-aches, hazy vision, lack of physical and mental co-ordination; many other sensations are similar to those familiar after the intake of too much alcohol. The higher one rises the more severe these conditions become; usually consciousness is lost at about 20,000ft, indicating that death resulting from anoxia, a total lack of oxygen, is near. In rarefied air the only way to increase the partial pressure of oxygen in the lungs is to inhale pure oxygen. As these medical facts came to be understood, so special supplies of oxygen were carried in balloons flying to any great height, and by the end of the nineteenth century this had become the norm.

A flying machine that merely drifted around the atmosphere at the whim of nature was not everyone's idea of a satisfactory one. Henri Giffard was the first person to obtain directional control in a lighter-than-air craft when in 1852 he attained a speed of 5mph by using the powers of a steam engine attached to an airship. In less than fifty years after that Count von Zeppelin was launching the first of his famous gigantic airships; and in 1901 Alberto Santos-Dumont, the dapper son of a wealthy Brazilian coffee planter, negotiated his dirigible round the Eiffel Tower in under thirty minutes to take home a prize of 125,000 francs. Although Santos-Dumont often executed hair-raising flights, many a time scraping the Paris rooftops in his dirigible, he always ascended immaculately dressed, wearing a boater, a bow tie and a carnation in his buttonhole, as if prepared to descend into the midst of the smartest Parisian garden party.

The development of the aeroplane

Man had overcome the law of gravity by using lighter-than-air craft that relied on a supply of hot air or hydrogen, and by the addition of an engine he was able to direct his craft; he had learnt about the lift that wings could produce so now he could also dangle from or perch on a powerless aeroplane, leap off a suitable hill and glide for hundreds of feet. But he was still unable to make an aeroplane which would take off under its own power and sustain its own flight. The American scientist, Professor Langley, and many others, were ridiculed for devoting their energies to this task. At the beginning of 1903 an editorial in the *New York Times* pompously proclaimed:

> The flying machine which will really fly might be evolved by the combined and continuous efforts of mathematicians and mechanicians in from one to ten million years – provided we can meanwhile eliminate such little drawbacks and embarrassments as the existing relation between weight and strength in inorganic materials. No doubt the problem has its attractions for those it interests, but to ordinary men, it would seem as if the effort might be employed more profitably.

The writer of those words might deservedly have found himself unemployed a few months later, when Orville and Wilbur Wright triumphed with the first controlled flight of a powered heavier-than-air craft. Three years later, in 1906, Santos-Dumont was officially proclaimed as the first person in Europe to fly a powered heavier-than-air craft. In November of that year he succeeded in flying his bizarre '14 bis' 722ft in twenty-one seconds – a speed of approximately twenty-five mph.

Wilbur Wright was a great catalyst to aeronautical advance in Europe when he visited France in 1908, making a series of public flights. In September he flew for almost twenty minutes, covering sixteen and a half miles; he captured the imagination of France and became a great hero. The admiration was obviously one-sided, for he dismissed the efforts of French aviators: 'My contract here in France stipulates that I should fly, not hop from the ground, or flutter along like a hen chased by a dog.' European efforts un-deniably appeared quite feeble by comparison to the Wrights' epic flights. By January 1908 a European aircraft had flown for one and a half minutes; whereas by the end of the same year Wilbur Wright had sustained a flight for two hours twenty minutes, and on many occasions had also taken up passengers.

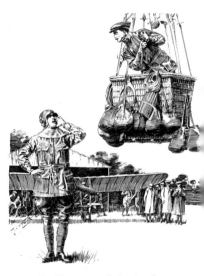

**Balloon and Aeroplane
Gabardine Burberry Outrigs**

It was the year 1909 that was marked by aeronautical successes. Blériot crossed the Channel in July, and the first great aviation meeting was held at Reims, attended by all the best pilots and manufacturers of the day as well as by thousands of spectators. Gradually, too, the rest of Europe was waking up to the fact that aviation was here to stay and that it had a great potential. Over the following five years air displays and aviation meetings were organised all over Europe and America, from Brussels and Budapest to Blackpool and Boston. People travelled miles to see their favourite aviators set up

M. Blériot in his flying boiler suit, July 1909.

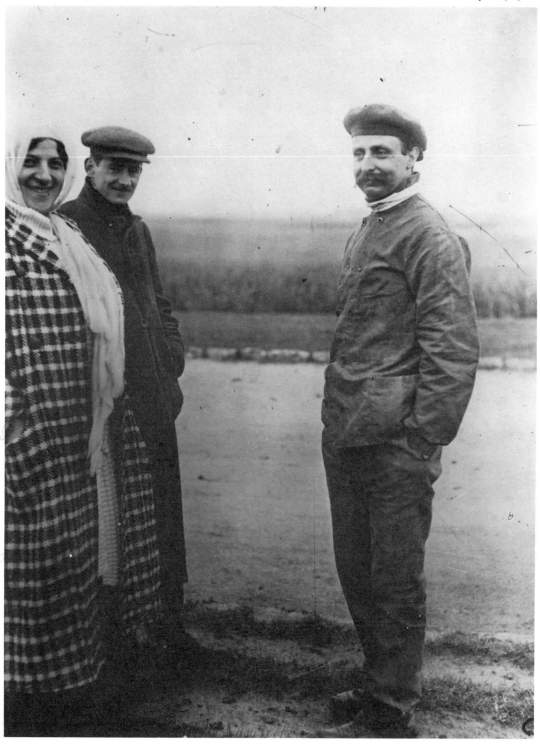

new records. The *Daily Mail* offered a £10,000 prize for the first flight from London to Manchester, Gordon Bennett put up a trophy for an annual speed contest, and Jacques Schneider established a seaplane speed contest for which he donated the famed Schneider Trophy. Furthermore, long-distance air races were becoming increasingly popular. These included the Circuit of Britain and Circuit of Europe, as well as daredevil flights from Paris to Rome or Cairo.

The first decade of powered flight was one of very great achievement. By 1914 aircraft were able to travel at over 100 mph, they could sustain their flight for hundreds of miles rather than a few hundred yards, and in December 1913 the French aviator Legagneux flew on his Nieuport monoplane to over 20,000 ft when for the first time oxygen was used in an aeroplane.

The development of controllable heavier-than-air craft in the first decade of the twentieth century meant an increase in speed and a resulting exposure to slipstream which had never been encountered in balloons and only slightly in airships. Miss Gertrude Bacon describes the sensations of aerial locomotion in an article in the *Aero* magazine of 1910:

> A flight in an aeroplane, in my own experience, is a time of stress and strain. It is cold, bitter cold, even on a sultry summer evening, for the furious gale of the onward motion blows through and through you, and makes your eyes smart and reddens your nose. It is deafeningly noisy. When I climbed down from the little basket seat of the Farman biplane that night at Reims the voices of Sommer and his mechanics sounded to my deadened ears as if they came from an immense distance away, and not for several minutes did I hear properly again.
>
> An hour's voyage by flying machine would, even for a passenger, make a not inconsiderable demand on bodily strength and nervous energy. But, oh! the rapturous thrill of the swift plunge through air, the glorious exhilaration of the swooping flight, the sense that never until that moment have you felt what it is really to live!

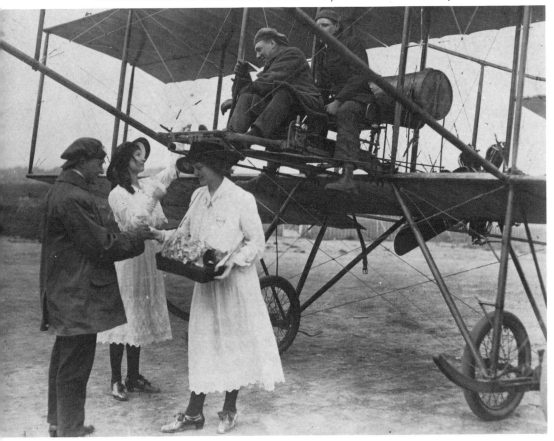

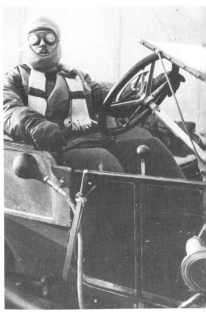

Aviators on Alexandra Rose Day. Note the reversed cloth caps.

Automobile attire; the ancestry of flying clothing is apparent.

Flying an early aeroplane, although on the whole a pastime for the rich, was certainly no comfortable affair. Perched on a hard little wicker seat, exposed to all the elements as well as the slipstream, one had to learn to withstand the bitter cold, the deafening roar of the engine, being splattered with oil, and the often unavoidable crash landings. Taking the slipstream into account, the rush of air encountered by the occupants of a tractor aircraft with an airspeed of sixty mph could be as much as ninety mph. The effects of propeller slipstream were, however, eliminated in a pusher biplane where the propeller was positioned to the rear of the aircraft. Many aviators were extremely wary of unstable meteorological conditions and in the early days would consider taking to the air only if their cigarette smoke rose vertically, whereas the more audacious pilot was prepared to encounter any adversity, including the weather.

Early aviators were dressed usually in their warmest underwear and tweeds, often adding a woollen balaclava, muffler and gloves for extra protection; doubtless the sort of clothing they would have donned for a spin in their automobile. When Blériot made his historic crossing of the Channel in the early morning of 25 July 1909 he wore his tweed suit, a khaki jacket lined with wool, a blue cotton boiler-suit on top to protect his tweeds from the splattering oil and a skull cap with ear flaps. This type of flying helmet later became known as a 'Blériot' helmet. He even had a pair of crutches strapped onto the fuselage as he had on two occasions recently badly burned his feet when the asbestos lining had come away from the aircraft's exhaust pipe. The trademark of a pilot was the traditional peaked cloth cap, reversed in order to prevent it from blowing off in mid-flight. Many an aspiring pilot would wander nonchalantly through the enclosure at an aviation meeting with his cap on back to front in the hope of gaining the admiring looks of the female spectators.

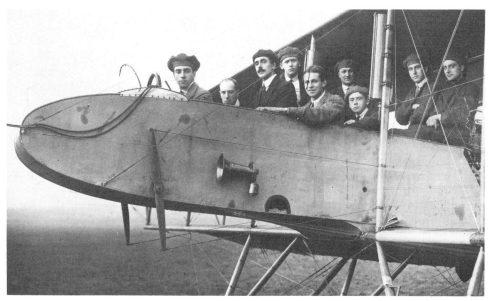

It is said that a few early French aviators who sported bristling moustaches were so vain that they felt it necessary to protect them in a metal container so that on landing the ladies would not be put off by any unsightly disarray! Etiquette was adhered to at all costs. It was not unusual in England for an aviator to dress up in his best suit, with a stiff white collar and bow tie. In America, Arch Hoxsey, a pilot in the Wright brothers' team and the Beau Brummel of American airmen, was reputed never to fly after 6 pm unless dressed in evening clothes. The American, Lincoln Beachey, was another of the individualist pioneer pilots who dressed primarily to please their public. He was famous for his flight in 1911 in a Curtiss aircraft over the Niagara Falls and under the nearby suspension bridge. He usually wore an extremely smart pin-striped suit with a high starched collar and diamond tiepin, but occasionally he chose to dress up as a woman and would take off in an aircraft, careering through the sky with his skirt and bonnet flapping wildly in the wind.

Grahame-White and company in his Chara-banc. It seems that almost anyone could look like an aviator if he turned his cap back to front.

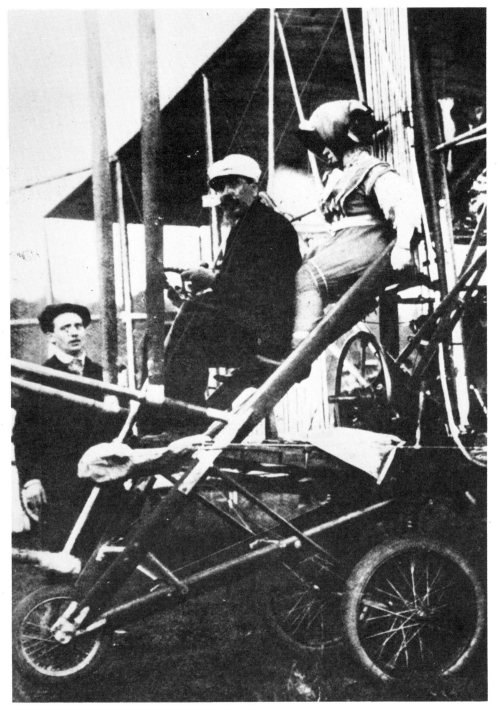

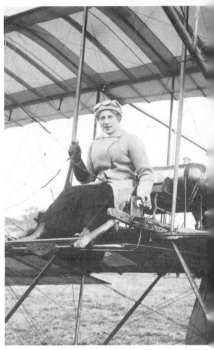

Mrs de Beauvoir Stocks, the second woman in Britain to get a pilot's licence.

Mr and Mrs Cody demonstrating the problems of open-cockpit flying.

Fashion problems

Needless to say, women found flying clothing a problem. In the early twentieth century it was considered highly improper to reveal any more than an ankle. But aeroplanes were breezy creatures, so, to prevent social disasters, women would often tie a rope just above their ankles. Mrs Hart O'Berg, the wife of the Wrights' business representative in Europe and the first woman passenger in an aeroplane, was taken aloft by Wilbur Wright in October 1908 and discovered this solution to the problem. She also tied a veil over her bonnet to keep her headgear secure.

The latest vogue in women's flying clothing was recorded in a contemporary magazine:

What to wear in the air no longer puzzles the birdwoman. Each woman flier has settled the matter to her satisfaction, and while the costumes may differ in detail to suit the individuality of the wearer there is sameness in the general outline.

The accepted toggery is a two-pice suit consisting of a blouse and knickerbockers and trouserettes. The headgear differs according to the feminine ideas. It may be an automobile cap or a becoming hood of some soft material.

Mlle Dutrieu, the French airwoman and the pioneer of her sex in the air, set a new fashion in flying clothes on her first appearance in this country at the Nassau Boulevard aerodrome. Her drab colored costume of cravenette serge caught the feminine eye as she swung across the flying field to give the spectators an idea of what a birdwoman looks like aground.

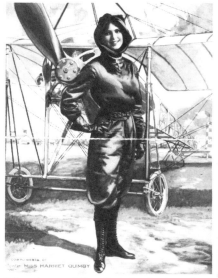

The elegant Miss Quimby in her plum-coloured costume.

Her two-piece suit consists of a blouse and a divided skirt, with a suggestion of the harem. The two garments are joined by a black patent leather belt and a Norfolk jacket effect is obtained by an arrangement sewed on the upper part of the skirt, which falls gracefully over the feet when she walks and with a button and strap is secured around her ankles before she mounts her Farman biplane.

The masculinity of her appearance is somewhat relieved by a small pair of patent leather boots topped with white. She wears an ordinary automobile cap.

Mlle Dutrieu is always corsetless when she soars. She says this affords freedom of movement and lessens the danger in case of a fall. Neither of the American fliers, Miss Quimby and Miss Moisant, takes this precaution.

Miss Harriet Quimby's plum-colored satin costume is perhaps more picturesque than that of Mlle Dutrieu. It has a blouse and knickerbockers with a monk hood attached. The knickerbockers have the inside seams closed by rows of buttons which when unfastened convert the knickers into a walking skirt. The blouse is cut with the long shoulder seams and fastens under the arm. Miss Quimby wears high-top leather boots.

She says her next costume will be plain knickerbockers, as she always wears a long coat when she is aground and there is no need of a skirt.

With the exception of the hood and the material the costume of Miss Moisant is practically a duplicate of the one worn by Miss Quimby. It is made of a heavy tan-colored cloth and inter-lined with silk, while Miss Quimby reverses the materials. Small patches of black net are inserted over the part of Miss Quimby's hood that covers the ears, so that she can keep in touch with the working of her engine.

Miss Quimby, who was the first woman to fly the Channel, explained in the American journal *Leslie's Weekly* how she

heeded Mr Hamel's warning about the coldness of the Channel flight and had prepared accordingly. Under my flying suit of wool-back satin I wore two pairs of silk combinations, over it a long woollen coat, over this an American raincoat, and around and across my shoulders a long wide stole of sealskin. Even this did not satisfy my solicitous friends. At the last minute they handed me up a large hot-water bag, which Mr Hamel insisted on tying to my waist like an enormous locket.

There was certainly a great variety of idiosyncratic and improvised clothing worn in the air. Some aviators donned their motoring clothing or adapted their warmest winter woolies for the occasion. But it was not much fun being soaked to the skin in a rain-storm or having the icy slipstream whistling up your flapping sleeve or trouser-leg. Incorrect clothing could be uncomfortable—indeed hazardous, as Claude Grahame-White, the famous British aviator, once discovered. He had a near disaster when desperately trying to catch up with his competitor in the London-to-Manchester air race of 1910. He courageously took to the air by night when suddenly his engine spluttered and faltered. Panic-stricken he fumbled with the invisible controls, only to discover that his sleeve had caught the ignition switch and turned it off. He flicked it on again and the engine roared back into life. Pilots also found it extremely troublesome attempting to locate and extricate their pocket watches. By 1912 according to a contributor to *Aeronautics* one of the aviator's characteristics was to wear his watch on a wrist strap.

The wise aviator soon began to realise that oil and dirt ruined his good tweed suit and that something more practical was necessary. Leading European stores, such as Gamages, Burberrys and Roold lost no time in meeting this new demand and started to manufacture aviators' combination suits, goggles, fleece-lined boots, rainproof gauntlets and leather coats. The deafening noise of the engine and slipstream could be reduced somewhat by the use of ear-bungs and leather flying helmets. Specialised flying clothing was advertised widely and became a must for most airmen. Paper underwear was put on the market as an aid to keeping warm. Unfortunately, its advertised qualities were not totally reliable as Georges Chavez, the Peruvian pilot, found to his cost. In September 1910 he entered a competition to fly across the Alps. This he achieved, but tragically crashed on landing. It seems likely that he was so numbed by the cold that he was unable to flatten his glide in time.

One of the great figures of early aviation i Britain Claude Grahame-White, in a Bur berry flying suit.

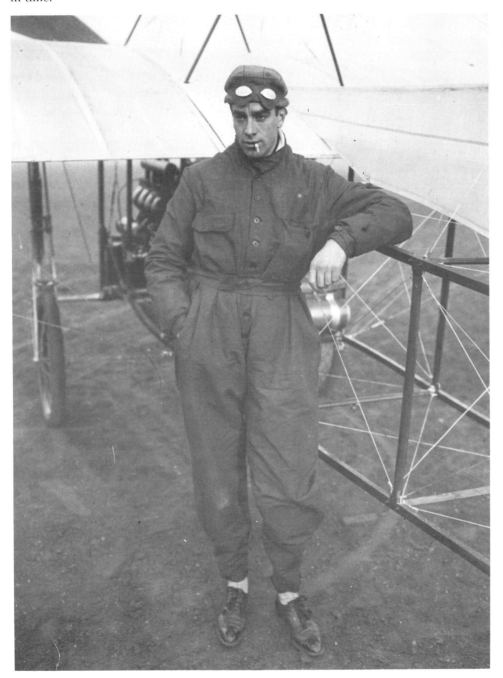

Goggles were produced in varying shapes and sizes, their manufacturers boasting different attributes. Adapted from motor-racing goggles, they prevented watering eyes and protected the eyes from dust and rain, for the most harmless raindrop becomes a stinging lash at sixty mph. When worn with the traditional cloth cap, goggles would often slip and proved difficult to take off without dislodging the cap. Dunhills therefore introduced the cloth cap with a flap at the back which incorporated the goggles. The aviator had only to lower the flap, reverse the cap, and the goggles were in position. Many early aircraft engines, including the air-cooled rotary Gnome and the Anzani engine of the Blériot XI, were noted for their propensity to throw oil all over the pilot, often bespattering his goggles and greatly impairing his vision. Commercial manufacturers did not attempt to solve this problem, but an improvised solution was to attach a wad of cotton to a piece of string dangling from the goggles, providing an accessible wiper when required. Non-flammable goggles were introduced, which reduced the danger of blindness in the ever-present risk of fire. Triplex brought some goggles on to the market with splinter-proof glass, thus greatly lessening the risk to the eyes. Chlorophyll glass was also used, allowing the aviator to fly against the most brilliant sunshine without being dazzled.

Pages of a catalogue produced by the famous French Clothing dealers 'Roold'.

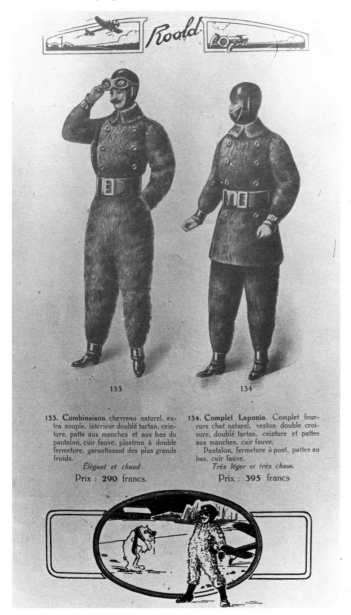

133. Combinaison chevreau naturel, extra souple, intérieur doublé tartan, ceinture, patte aux manches et aux bas du pantalon, cuir fauve, plastron à double fermeture, garantissant des plus grands froids.
Élégant et chaud.
Prix : 290 francs.

134. Complet Laponia. Complet fourrure chat naturel, veston double croisure, doublé tartan, ceinture et pattes aux manches, cuir fauve.
Pantalon, fermeture à pont, pattes au bas, cuir fauve.
Très léger et très chaud.
Prix : 395 francs

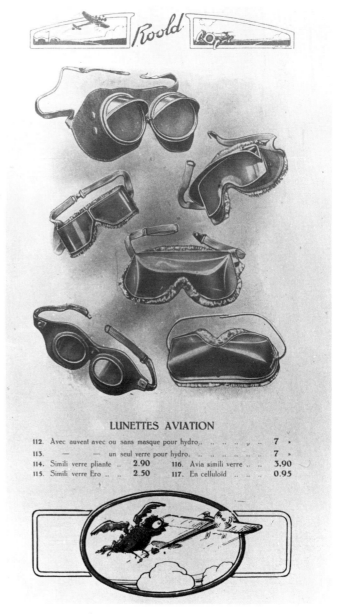

LUNETTES AVIATION

112.	Avec auvent avec ou sans masque pour hydro.			7 .
113.	— — un seul verre pour hydro.			7 »
114.	Simili verre pliante ..	2.90	116. Avia simili verre	3.90
115.	Simili verre Ero	2.50	117. En celluloïd	0.95

Ideally, flying clothing should not only be warm, comfortable and practical, but it should also, wherever possible, safeguard the physical well-being of the pilot in case of accident. In the early days aircraft were essentially unpredictable and unreliable. Pilot training was hardly thorough–one learnt by trial and error–and crash-landings were a commonplace hazard. The principles of flight were not properly understood, and to many the stall was inexplicable and always fatal. One was lucky to get away with a few bumps and bruises on returning to earth.

As with today's controversy about the advantages of wearing seat belts in cars, so in the early years of this century a similar battle raged in the aviation world. Many considered that it was better to be thrown clear of a crash than to be trapped by a seat belt or harness inside the wreckage. But three tragedies were to lend support to the alternative view, for in November 1910 Ralph Johnstone, a member of the Wright brothers' exhibition team, was killed at Denver, Colorado. One account of the accident stated that in a poorly executed tight turn he was thrown from his seat. He frantically grabbed the controls to save himself, exerting too much 'G'. As a result of this, the aircraft's wing structure collapsed. A similar disaster befell Harriet Quimby, the first woman to gain a

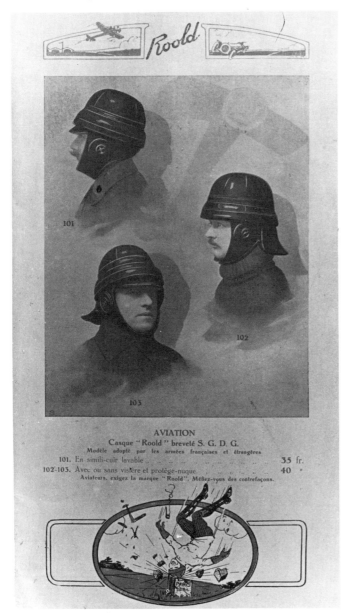

AVIATION
Casque "Roold" breveté S. G. D. G.
Modèle adopté par les armées françaises et étrangères
101. En simili-cuir lavable . . . . 35 fr.
102-103. Avec ou sans visière et protège-nuque . . . . . 40 "
Aviateurs, exigez la marque "Roold". Méfiez-vous des contrefaçons.

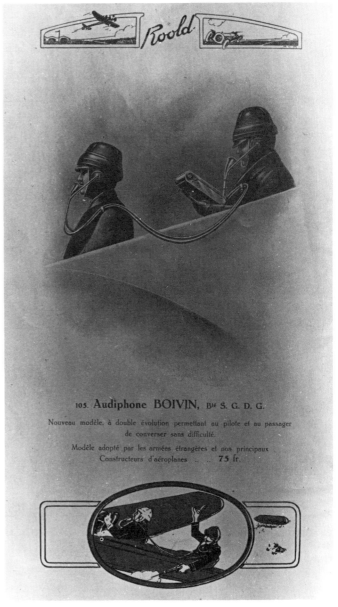

105. Audiphone BOIVIN, Bté S. G. D. G.
Nouveau modèle, à double évolution permettant au pilote et au passager de converser sans difficulté.
Modèle adopté par les armées étrangères et nos principaux Constructeurs d'aéroplanes . . 75 fr.

pilot's licence in America and the first female to fly the English Channel. Taking part in an aviation meet at Boston in 1912 her Blériot monoplane was caught in turbulent air and she and her passenger were thrown clear of the aircraft, plumetting 1,000 ft to their deaths in the sea beneath. A year later Colonel Cody and a passenger were killed when they fell from their aircraft after it had begun to break up in mid-air. Cody was superstitious and refused to fly with anyone wearing anything green. He would never have taken to the air on this occasion if he had known that his passenger was wearing green socks.

Fatal injuries often occurred if the pilot was not strapped in, for on crashing or landing heavily or, as we have seen, if the aircraft was thrown around the skies, the pilot could be thrown forward into the instrument panel, or be pitched out altogether. The latter was especially so with the Wright biplane and the Henry Farman, in which the pilot was perched on a small seat on the leading edge of the plane with no protection at all in front of him. The situation was particularly grave if the aircraft turned turtle. The dangers were slightly reduced when aircraft designers such as Voisin and Maurice Farman began to protect their pilots in a basic form of nacelle, and the addition of skids helped to cushion the shock. The Antoinette and REP were both sensibly equipped with rudimentary seat belts. A writer in the *Aeroplane* of 1911 spoke for an increasing body of opinion: 'There is no particular objection to a man breaking himself if he really wishes to do so, but when he has a lingering prejudice in favour of remaining in one piece it is sheer foolishness of him not to take even the simplest precautions.' The only criticism of the early seat belt was that it was rigid, and on impact either snapped or else, remaining intact, inflicted internal injuries on the pilot; but by 1911 elasticised straps were introduced as well as quick-release mechanisms.

Mr Warren wearing a helmet of his invention takes a flying leap at the hangar to demonstrate the helmet's utility.

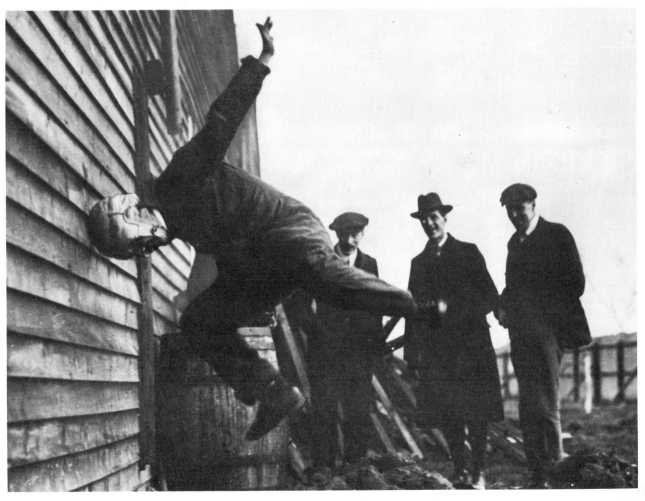

Other safety accessories developed at this time included hard crash or safety helmets which were developed from motor-cycle racing helmets; though practical, however, they were not especially popular. *Flight* of March 1912 wrote:

> How seldom it is one sees an aviator wearing a safety helmet these days! For this, the reason is rather difficult to define, unless it be that, in common with others, aviators dislike to be reminded of the risks they are running, however small they may be. Nevertheless, many aviators at the present day owe their lives to the use of safety helmets. Safety helmets may be rather unsightly to wear, but are not goggles equally unlovely?

Mr Warren in his helmet.

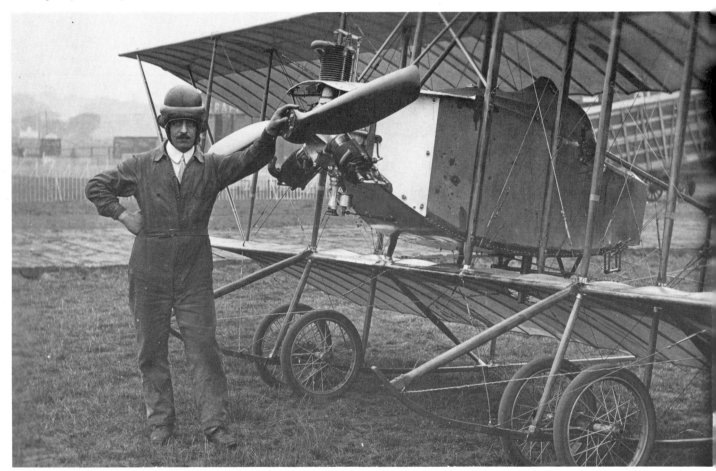

On the other hand the *Aeroplane* of October 1912 felt that it was the novices who failed to take the sensible precaution of protecting their heads for fear of being regarded as cowards by others. The article wisely concluded: 'More men are killed by moral cowardice than by physical.'

Establishments such as Roold in Paris and Brown and Dunhills in England, well known for their excellent motoring and flying clothing, began to manufacture safety helmets for aviators. The ubiquitous Mr Warren of Hendon produced a safety helmet which bears his name. He was even prepared to demonstrate its strength by flinging himself head first against a wall, and by letting his fellow-mechanics thump him on the head with hammers. The Warren helmet had excellent shock-absorbing qualities and was widely used by many airmen.

Yet another worthwhile safety precaution was wearing a life-jacket for flights over water. Many aviators came to grief through neglecting this, for in water flying clothes soon became waterlogged and extremely heavy. Cork belts were frequently worn, as were inflated tyre tubes, but these accessories were all rather cumbersome. In 1913 a French firm introduced the Perrin Arm-Brace which they claimed was 'as a lifeboat in one's pocket and will allow you in case of shipwreck or accident, to float while waiting for help, and also to save and rescue your neighbour if needed.' The reviewer in the *Aeroplane* pertinently remarked, 'Oh, Mr Perrin, is it that you are a wag, or only a pessimisanthropist?' The arm-brace was a rubberised air-bag with the appearance of a waistcoat. It could be inflated immediately by releasing a small 'sparklets' tube of compressed air into the airtight bag. Unlike conventional life-saving equipment the arm-brace, the precursor of the Mae West, was quite comfortable and unobtrusive and yet could be readily inflated in time of emergency.

Life-jackets and parachutes will not be dealt with in detail in this book for, strictly speaking, they are part of one's survival equipment rather than flying clothing; however, they are worn by the pilot in flight and inasmuch as they greatly increase a pilot's life expectancy in case of emergency, their presence is a psychological reassurance which allows the pilot to concentrate more on controlling the aircraft. Parachutes were developed for balloonists at the end of the eighteenth century and were used by military observers on many occasions. The balloonist wore a harness and when he leapt out of the basket the shroud lines attached to the harness pulled the silk chute from its canvas container which was fastened to the outside of the basket. An American, A. L. Stevens, as early as 1908, invented a free-type parachute operated manually by the wearer, but this was not developed until after World War I.

The intrepid Mr W. Newall about to make the first parachute descent from an aeroplane in Great Britain. May 1914.

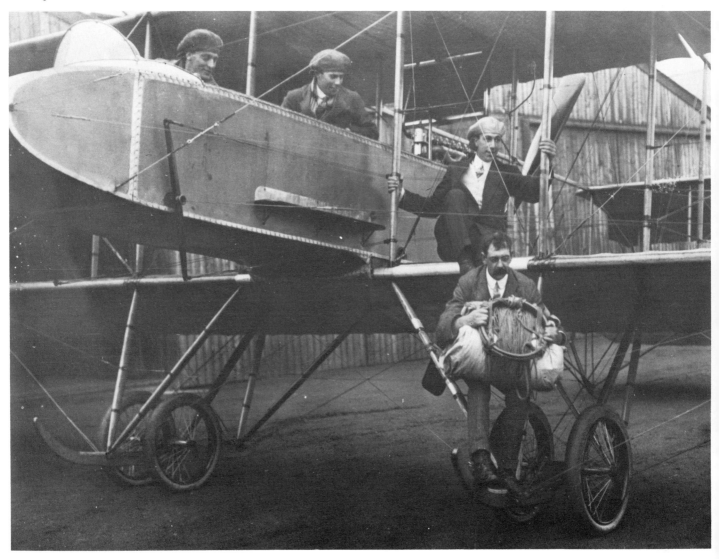

In a lighter vein the *Aeroplane* offered advice on safety precautions:

> Never let your beard grow long. It may so easily become entangled in the propeller.
> False teeth are best left at home in the strongbox: engine vibration is apt to dislodge them.
> And, above all things, bear in mind that Dr Gimbell's Glutinous Globules are death to airsickness.

By 1912 flying was no longer regarded solely as an exhilarating sport. The shadow of war was creeping across Europe, gradually awakening officialdom to the possible role aeroplanes could play in warfare. The War Office had accepted the potential of lighter-than-air craft as early as 1878 when experiments with observation balloons were carried out at Woolwich. Later that year the War Office allocated £150 for the construction of a balloon designed by Captain J. L. B. Templer, who was to become the chief ballooning instructor to the Corps of Royal Engineers. In the early 1880s the Balloon Equipment Store was moved from Woolwich to Chatham, thence to Aldershot, and in 1905 it moved to South Farnborough, a place associated in those early days with pioneers such as the indefatigable Mr S. F. Cody, the Chief Kiting Instructor, and Colonel J. E. Capper. The Royal Engineers from the Balloon Section used to ascend in free and tethered balloons wearing their dashing red and blue serge uniforms, which appeared to provide adequate protection against the chilly atmosphere at observation heights.

The great Mr S. F. Cody in his suit, thigh-length riding boots and a Gamages helmet astride his 'Cathedral' biplane for the military trials on Salisbury Plain. 1912.

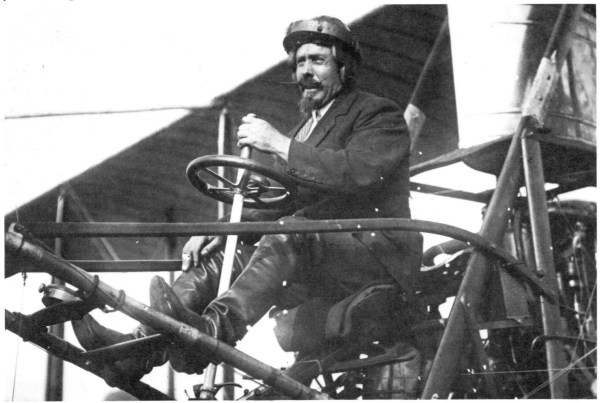

It was Colonel Capper who in 1908 directed the first successful ground-to-air wireless telegraphy communications. Radio was still in its infancy but messages in Morse could be received in a balloon, and from balloons as far afield as twenty miles. Two years later the actor Robert Loraine transmitted a wireless message in Morse from a Bristol Boxkite to the nearby Larkhill experimental ground station, becoming the first man in Britain to transmit a message from an aeroplane in flight. Further experiments continued at Brooklands, the main problem being that of engine noise. It was not, however, until the war years that the Morse messages of wireless telegraphy were superseded by the verbal messages of radio telephony.

Although the balloon had been adopted by the War Office, heavier-than-air craft were regarded with scepticism by the British Government, and progress tended to be hampered by the conventional, wary attitudes of those in command. As late as 1910 the British Secretary of State for War declared, 'We do not consider that aeroplanes will be of any possible use for war purposes,' yet in the following year the Air Battalion of the Royal Engineers was formed consisting of one company of airships, one of man-lifting kites used for reconnaissance purposes, one of balloons and another of aeroplanes. The Government had obviously realised that in wartime it could be advantageous to fly over the enemy, observe their size and movements and report one's discoveries back to base. The Balloon School at Farnborough now became known as the Army Aircraft Factory and £85,000 was allocated for the development of dirigibles and aeroplanes.

The Air Battalion of the Royal Engineers, consisting of fourteen officers and 176 NCOs, decided that the former must be readily distinguishable when in flying clothing and proposed the wearing of a leather jacket onto which would be attached shoulder straps and rank badges. Bedford cord service dress breeches were to be discarded in favour of leather breeches since the former would 'not keep out the wind when travelling at forty miles an hour'. Loose leggings were also to be worn, lined with lambswool and reaching from the calf to the thigh. Other accessories to guard against cold and dirt included gauntlets to prevent the wind from blowing up the sleeves, and a fur-lined cap which tied under the chin and kept the ears warm. No final decisions were in fact taken on the question of flying clothing for officers, as most men working in this field preferred to wear the traditional all-in-one boiler suit and 'Blériot'-type helmet.

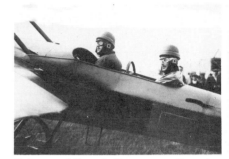

Prévost and Captain Dawes on a Deperdussin, sporting their safety helmets. 1912.

Events moved fast after the formation of the Air Battalion in 1911. In 1912 it was suggested that a single Flying Corps be established consisting of a military and naval wing and a Central Flying School at Upavon. The Royal Flying Corps, as it was then called, was planned to comprise seven squadrons, each squadron being equipped with twelve aircraft, with two pilots per aircraft. But there were only eight naval officers and eleven army officers who were qualified pilots, so it was obvious that a large-scale training programme had to be mounted. Unfortunately the efficiency of this unified air service was greatly impaired when, in July 1914, the Admiralty broke away and established its own Royal Naval Air Service; thus the country went to war with two separate air arms.

Pilots in the RFC and RNAS wore their everyday service dress uniforms for flying. For the former this consisted of a khaki serge, double-breasted jacket known as a 'maternity jacket', Bedford cord breeches, brown ankle-boots and khaki puttees. Pilots were permitted to wear a variety of commercially manufactured clothing for added warmth as there was as yet no official issue of flying clothing. Brown leather coats and jackets were worn, motorcyclist's gauntlets from the transport section, all sorts of brown leather flying helmets, countless designs of goggles and the popular, long woolly scarf patiently knitted at home by a loving mother, wife or girl friend.

The naval wing of the RFC, later the RNAS, similarly, wore their service dress of dark blue breeches, puttees, and single-breasted jacket as well as black ankle-boots. Very often it was necessary to add a white jersey and scarf and a heavy blue overcoat, as well as the vital leather flying helmet to reduce the cold and noise.

The last days of peace

Although aviation in its various forms was now accepted as part of military and naval life its role was restricted by an inbred scepticism of innovations and a fear that powers long held by the army and navy would be usurped. The idea of using aviation in an offensive role was widely mistrusted, and so aircraft were allocated the limited job of reconnaissance and observation in time of war. Military commanders had had every opportunity to see the excellent capabilities of aircraft: in 1912 and 1913 air displays were held every two weeks at Hendon. Flour bags simulating bombs were dropped on the outline of a battleship to prove that aerial bombing was a perfectly feasible proposition. In 1912 Claude Grahame-White initiated a 'Wake Up England' campaign claiming, 'the object of this display is to educate the people of this country as to the qualities and potentialities of the 'new arm' and to stimulate the Government and the War Office to

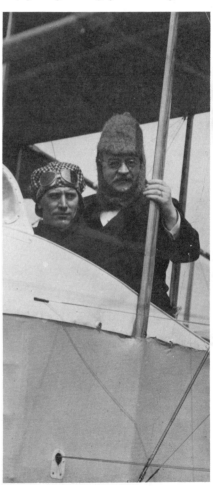

The time has come, the walrus said . . . ! The Lord Mayor of Manchester, Alderman McCabe, the first Lord Mayor to take to the air. He is flying with Verrier from Trafford Park.

make good the deficiency caused by past neglect.' He flew to many parts of England in an earnest bid to achieve this aim.

When war broke out in August 1914 Britain had far fewer military aircraft than Germany. In fact a mere handful of aircraft was able to cross the Channel and join the British Expeditionary Force in France. For economic reasons the War Office had turned to its own Royal Aircraft Factory at Farnborough, a descendant of the Army Aircraft Factory, for the design and construction of aircraft. This institution had been impeded by lack of finance and encouragement from the Government, but in 1911 a talented team led by F. M. Green and Geoffrey de Havilland designed the BE1, the first practical military aircraft. This tractor biplane could attain a speed of fifty-nine mph with two passengers, and was holder of the altitude record for a British heavier-than-air craft. The BE1 and BE2 were to emerge in the early days of the war as the BE2c, one of the most successful reconnaissance aircraft of the period.

In 1913 A. V. Roe built his Avro 504 biplane. This two-seater tractor aircraft was a typical military machine of the immediate pre-war period. It had a speed range of between thirty-five and eighty-two mph and was to render valuable service as a bomber, fighter and reconnaissance aircraft, as well as being used as a standard trainer until 1933. The pilot was protected to a considerable extent from the hazards of cold, as well as from crash landings, by being able to sit in a cockpit integrated into the fuselage or nacelle. No longer did he have to perch uncomfortably on a wicker seat balanced precariously on the lower mainplane.

Until the 1930s passengers and pilot alike were subjected to the unpleasant effects of slipstream, cold and rain. More protection was undoubtedly gained, for example, if one was sitting in an Avro-type of aircraft rather than on a Bristol Boxkite, but the real solution lay in an enclosed cockpit. This development was not to be put into general use for another two decades, but was foreshadowed by the designs of A. V. Roe who, in 1912, constructed an Avro cabin monoplane and biplane. In the same year Blériot designed an aircraft with an open cockpit for the pilot, and enclosed cabin for passengers. Amazing progress was also being made in Russia, where in 1912 Sikorsky built a huge multi-engined biplane known as Le Grand. He felt that the pilot should be assisted by a navigator and mechanics and that all should be in a large enclosed cabin to protect them from the bitter Russian weather. Sikorsky was possibly one of the first aircraft designers fully to appreciate that an uncomfortable pilot cannot perform his duties satisfactorily. The pilot's enclosed compartment was fitted with dual controls, had excellent visibility and full standing room. A balcony linked this area with the passenger cabin which had four seats, a sofa and table, and a lavatory in the rear. Le Grand's successor, the Ilia Mourometz, which first flew in December 1913, boasted electric light supplied by a wind-driven generator and heat from two pipes through which passed part of the exhaust. It could also carry sixteen passengers. This precocious aircraft was undoubtedly the first forerunner of the modern airliner. By enclosing and heating the cabins of both pilot and passengers Sikorsky largely eliminated the need to wear innumerable layers of bulky clothing.

By 1914 the aviation world had clearly come to appreciate that the dangers of flying an aircraft were multiplied if the pilot's powers of concentration were in any way impaired. When exposed to the inclemencies of the weather in a bone-shaking, noisy, dirty aircraft it was vital to be cocooned in layers of warm, comfortable clothing. It was obviously extremely dangerous for a pilot to have to spend his time frantically shaking his wrists, wriggling his toes and earnestly praying that the sickness of cold would disappear, rather than concentrating fully on the control of the aircraft. But although aviators did all they could to overcome these hazards most aircraft designers were too heavily involved with the basic enigmas of aerodynamics to be able to devote any more than secondary importance to the comfort of the pilot.

It was with such problems largely unsolved that in August 1914 Europe was plunged into war, and aircraft that were still in their infancy were forced to play a major role in the ensuing holocaust.

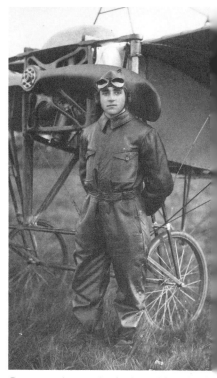

Desoutter, immaculately dressed in a leather flying suit. Note the helmet with rolls of leather by the ears to deflect the air and reduce the noise.

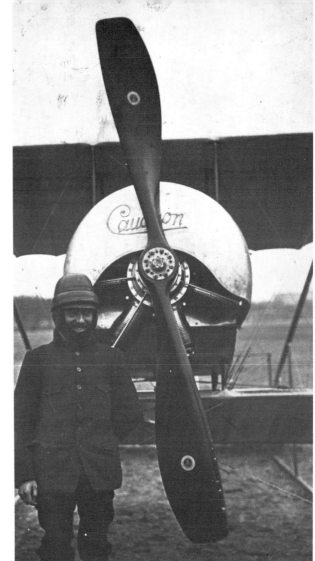

Chantel in a Roold helmet.

Smile please! Howard Pixton at Hendon.
Note the wrist altimeter.

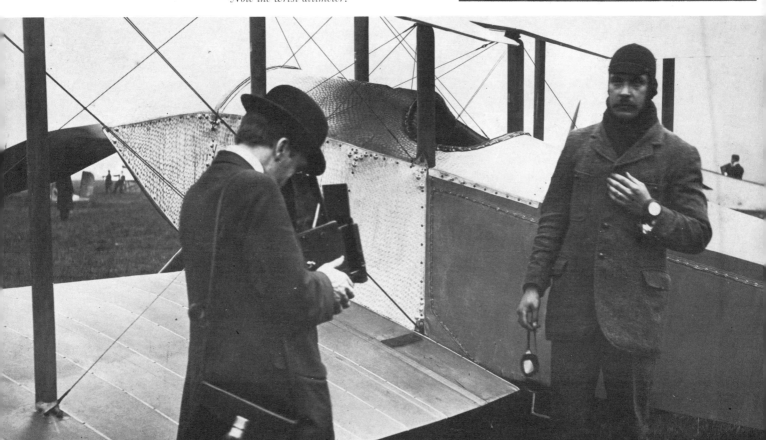

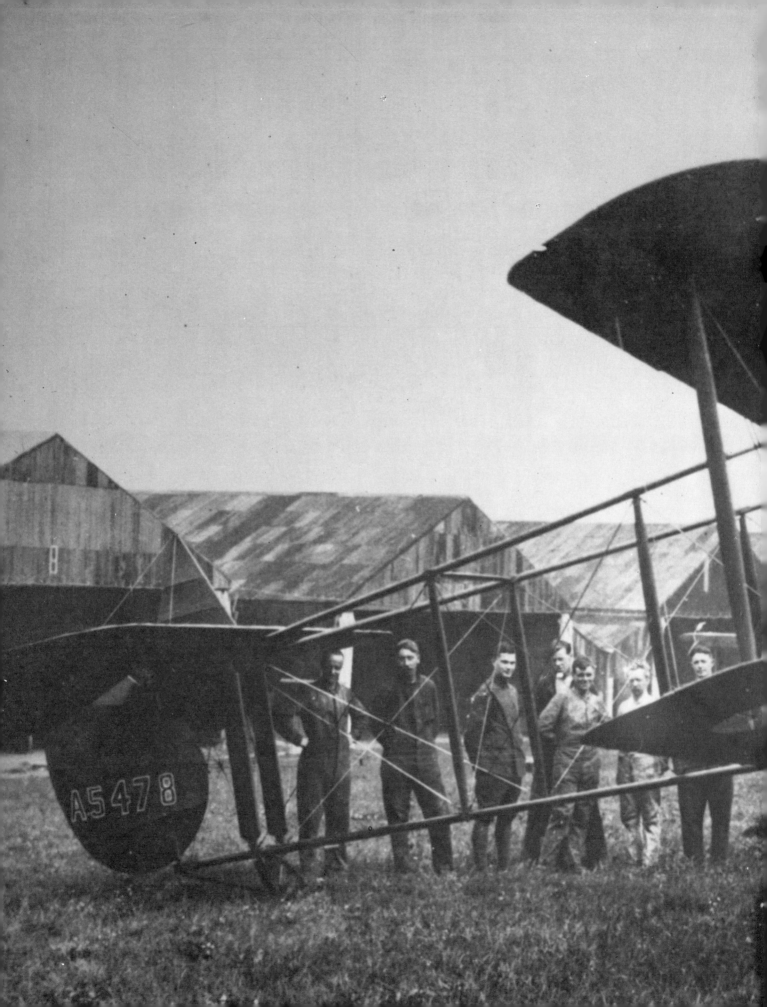

CHAPTER 2
KNIGHTS OF THE AIR 1914–18

GOLD COAST No 10

From the peaceful flying fields of Upavon, Brooklands, Hendon and many more, military aviators began their training, successfully acquired their pilot's brevets and became flying members of those two services, the Royal Flying Corps and the Royal Naval Air Service. To these men the perils of sustained flight were still to come. The intensity of their early training can be understood when an announcement reading, 'Beatty School of Flying, Wright biplanes 40, 50 and 60 horse-power, also Handley Page 50 horse-power monoplane, dual controls for easy instruction, all flights last 15 minutes in winds up to 20 miles per hour, tuition fee £75,' was just typical of a school advertisement. A commission in one of the flying services was also open to civilians with officer potential who, if they learnt to fly privately, could obtain a Royal Aero Club certificate and join the Special Reserve.

The war which started in August 1914 would need men, and up to then flying men had been rare, despite the training offered to all ranks of the RNAS and RFC in the two preceding years. The supply of properly trained men and the development of equipment were to become the great problems for the flying services in the next four years.

At the outbreak of war aircraft types were numerous but not too efficient; an age of rapid development with great technical advances was about to begin. Aircraft designers knew very little about aerodynamics, far less about the military potential of their designs. The RFC intended to use aircraft for reconnaissance purposes, a field of military aviation in which the aircraft had, in military manoeuvres, already proved itself. This role did not necessitate any major changes in the design of existing aircraft, such as the BE2 series of biplanes, which were at this time eminently suitable as observation platforms. Small bombs could be carried and dropped from these machines, but the main objective was to report the enemy's movements. The RNAS, seeing more strategic advantages in the aeroplane, patronised companies like Short and Sopwith, and by the outbreak of war were purchasing aircraft that could play an offensive role, using bombs, torpedoes and guns. In the months and years to come both services would come to use and develop aircraft for defensive as well as offensive purposes.

The Army and Navy used motorised transport so their motoring garments were offered to pilots. In the early days motoring was an exposed and active outdoor pursuit and had already run up against the problems of weather and slipstream. A variety of garments had been devised to make life for the motorist more bearable. Goggles kept wind, dust and insects from the eyes and were worn with the balaclava, or the smarter leather, helmet. Gauntlets and a variety of weatherproof coats were also available. These articles worn over or with a uniform gave a fair degree of protection against the elements when flying. However, many airmen preferred and were allowed to purchase their own protective clothing rather than wear what was offered to them by the RFC or RNAS. Commercial companies had launched into the field of flying clothing and widely advertised flying hel-helmets, overalls and coats as well as an extensive range of accessories such as goggles, ear-bungs and gauntlets. Throughout the war companies like Burberrys, Gamages and Pride and Clark, advertised and sold garments in wool, leather and materials such as gabardine to members of the RFC and RNAS. Names like the Tie Locken Coat, patented by Burberrys, became famous on the Western Front.

But the trademark of wartime RFC aircrews was the brown chrome-leather coat. These coats were of knee length, flapped or double-breasted with buttons and had a belt and three pockets, including one on the left breast for maps. Fur collars were not issued, but many men had their coats modified to suit their personal requirements. A seeming luxury, fur collars could become extremely undesirable when sodden by rain and frozen by intense cold. Although these coats were official issue and bore the WD stamp, commercial companies produced and advertised identical garments, in black for the RNAS and brown for the RFC. This fact makes it impossible to ascertain from a photograph whether the wearer purchased his coat or had it issued to him. Thigh-length, sheepskin-lined boots known as 'fug'-boots were also widely used by British aircrews in World War I.

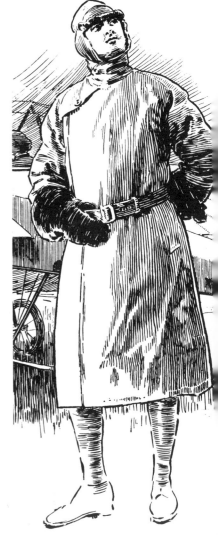

Burberrys' Air Kit supplies warmth whilst avoiding weight, by means of the finest and densest weaving, in conjunction with the thickest and lightest of linings.

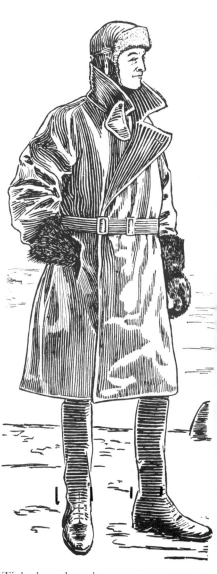

Tielocken has become synonymous with comfort. Its simplicity of adjustment together with the way its double fronts defy cold, gladdens the heart of the Airman.

Advances in air warfare

The guns of August thundered the 'war to end all wars' into the fields and hedgerows of France and Belgium. Eager and equipped, the German army was on the move. On 13 August 1914 the first aerial armada of the British Expeditionary Force (BEF) stood ready. Aeroplanes assembled from the RFC resources were the most advanced types available and were gathered at great sacrifice. From Dover thirty-seven aircraft took off, bound for France, on 14 August. Each pilot was given a revolver, field glasses, a spare pair of goggles, a small stove, a tin of biscuits, some cold meat, a piece of chocolate, soup cubes, and his orders. Those that successfully made the Channel crossing would carry out valuable work in the coming months. Squadrons were formed from reinforcements and a supply chain was set up. The long years of reconnaissance flights began. And as if flying an aeroplane was not difficult and hazardous enough, the length of time spent in the air was now increased. The first reconnaissance flight over enemy lines was carried out by Captain Joubert de la Ferté of No 3 Squadron, flying a Blériot XI, and Lieutenant G. W. Mapplebeck of No 4 Squadron in a BE2 on 19 August. Activity increased rapidly, for on 22 August no less than twelve flights were made. During one of these flights Sergeant-Major D. S. Jillings of No 2 Squadron was wounded in the leg by rifle fire from the ground. He was the first flying victim of the war.

*Shorthorn instructor and pupil.
An RFC pilot at St Omer, 1914. Over his uniform he wears an RFC issue short leather flying coat and fur lined helmet.*

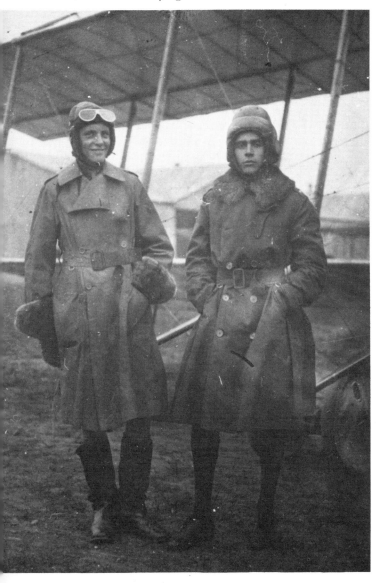

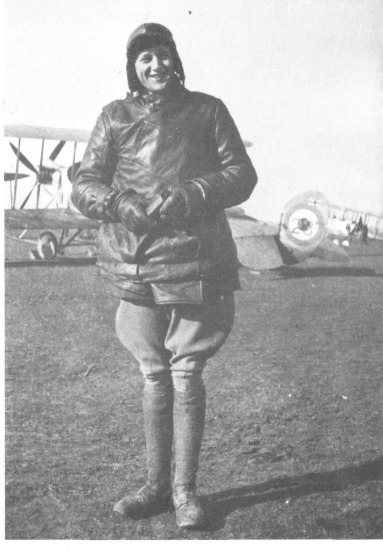

Fighting men for centuries have developed means of protection against their foes; a new weapon stimulates a new means of personal defence. The splendid attire of medieval knights epitomised the age of personal armour bearing heraldic devices. Larger numbers of combatants had of necessity reduced the individual glamour, uniformity taking its place. Such was the state that existed in France in 1914. With the special problems of flight a new, and often very tatty, form of external armour was in use. Well-worn, oily and scarred attire would soon be considered a mark of the wearer's prowess and experience in the air.

The aviator's enemies were the elements and his own inexperience; the bullet and shell had not effectively been taken into account. The steel helmet of the infantry man was rarely worn in an aeroplane. Warren and Roold leather-padded crash helmets were common, and used primarily to protect the wearer against his own failings in a bad landing accident. Helmets also gave the wearers relief from engine and slipstream noise. Nearly all soft-leather helmets had rolls of leather in front of the ears to help reduce noise, although this arrangement was obviously not particularly effective as many pilots bought wax-impregnated, cotton wool ear-bungs. The primary aim of the aviator's clothing was to protect him from the bitter cold and crash landings rather than from the bullet.

In the course of spotting gun and enemy positions, pilots found themselves fired at by ground troops as well as by anti-aircraft shellfire, affectionately called 'Archie', which followed the lazily circling aircraft on their errands. Over the lines, Allied and enemy aircraft encounters often involved the pilots, if their machines were evenly matched for speed, flying alongside each other and, firing revolvers or rifles and dropping small bombs or grenades on each other from above. None of these methods met with much success, though the seeds of aerial aggression were being sown. Harassing raids with small bombs were found by both sides to be desirable and a certain amount of official notice resulted.

The war would not be over in a week. Already hundreds of thousands of troops had died on the ground; men in enemy observation aircraft had helped to ensure this. Men were dying in the air too. Crashes and the occasional lucky shot all helped, and as a result efforts were made to enlist more men to maintain the growing strength of the flying

Some of the helmets and face protectors used in World War I were of rather bizarre appearance.

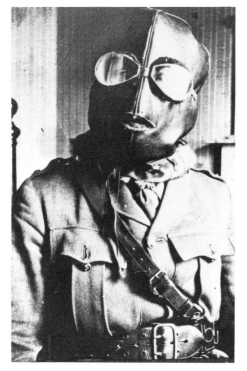 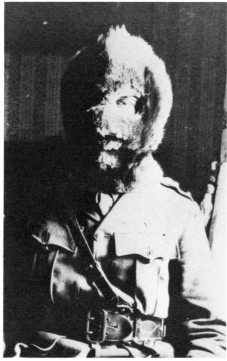 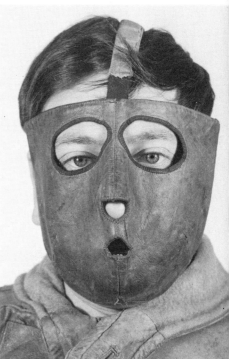

services. By 11 September 1914 the age limit for holders of the Royal Aero Club Pilot's Certificate had been significantly dropped from eighteen to seventeen. The number of certificates issued by December 1914 was still only 1,002. Many of those pilots were not actually in military service; a few were engaged in test flying and ferry work. Mr C. Gordon Bell was recorded by *Flight*, while test flying at Hendon, as wearing an interesting clothing innovation, a soft-leather face mask with eye-holes. This contrasted sinisterly with his peaked cap and tweed suit. When developed by manufacturers like Dunhills this device became quite common on the Western Front and doubtless saved the youthful complexion of its wearers.

Throughout the summer of 1914 the RFC had given important information to High Command, which averted disasters at Mons and the Battle of the Marne. The exceptional summer of 1914 turned to bitter winter. Flying continued despite appalling weather conditions through the first Battle of Ypres, where the war of mobility ended and trench warfare began. The first winter of the war saw the great armies in a position of stalemate. Lady Henderson, wife of the Commander-in-Chief of the RFC, organised the dispatch of clothing parcels to men of the RFC in an attempt to make Christmas more bearable. The woollen scarves, socks and mittens must have been welcomed and worn by all. Lady Henderson continued throughout the war to help men of the RFC.

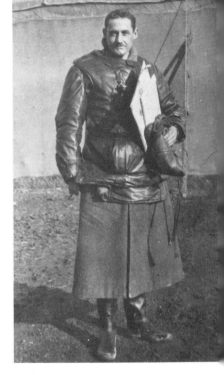

An observer at St Omer warmly dressed in double breasted short leather coat over an Army greatcoat, with a pair of binocular round his neck. 1914.

By bitter experience

Most of the flying in the early years of the war was at or below 3,000 ft. It could be cold, wet and rough for the pilots. Heights of 8,000–12,000 ft were sometimes achieved, but for most pilots in the active war zone this sort of height impeded observation of the enemy. To supplement the rudimentary instruments in an aircraft of this period pilots could, and did, buy altimeters of their own. The General Aeronautical Company sold pocket and wrist altimeters for £3. 17s. 6d., with dials normally reading up to 7,000 ft with an additional red section dealing with heights of from 8,000 to 10,000 ft. This product is ample testimony to the working heights of most aircraft. Zeppelin airships and Taube aircraft could fly at, and bomb, virtually unopposed, from the then considerable altitudes of 16,000 ft and more.

The German rigid airships made the first raids on the civilian population of the British Isles on 19 January 1915 when two Zeppelins attacked Yarmouth and King's Lynn. These machines flew for sustained periods at high altitudes. Flight Sub-Lieutenant R. A. J. Warneford brought down the first Zeppelin, LZ37, when he bombed it from his Morane Parasol aircraft. He had to climb to 11,000 ft before he was in range of the enemy airship. The cold was acute at this height and seriously hampered his attack, the only consolation being that for the Zeppelin crew conditions were no better, and they had to sustain their misery for much longer. Zeppelins had been fitted with oxygen equipment from the beginning of the war, something not yet contemplated by the British Forces, despite the use of breathing equipment by pioneer balloonists for many years. However, British coastal airships were not intended to operate at high altitudes as they had to remain in contact with the fleets and convoys for which they acted as watch-dogs. Captain Meager, who flew in these early airships, writes, 'Crews often wore the "Submarine Frock", a roomy hand-knitted sweater. A warm and comfortable article to wear when piloting was the naval "Lammy" coat, fixed by loops and toggles across the front. This coat had a hood which could be pulled tight around the head, keeping out rain, hail and snow; this worn over the "Submarine Frock" was very comfortable.' Thus attired the men of the RNAS patrolled the sea lanes for three years.

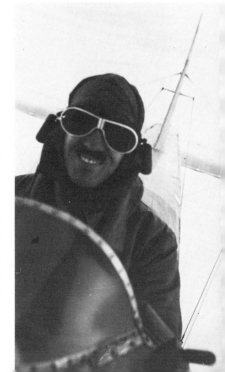

An airman secure in the knowledge that he i wearing Triplex safety goggles.

Whatever you chose to fly in on the Western Front, you could be reasonably certain of three things: as you went higher it became colder, that a prevailing south-westerly wind averaging twenty mph would usually be blowing, and that the sun would rise in the east and set in the west. Therefore to the RFC and French flying east, penetration across the enemy lines was rapid, but aircraft flying at seventy mph for some time over enemy territory would find themselves under prolonged enemy fire when tediously flogging home westwards. The sun added to the problems, as an RFC dawn patrol involved flying into the rising sun. Because of this patrols were preferred in the afternoon, whilst the Germans flew westwards on patrol at first light.

The following letter, written to Lady Henderson by her son Ian, who had just arrived at No 2 Squadron in France, gives the reader a good impression of life near the Front and how pilots equipped themselves.

No 2 Squadron
1st Wing
BEF

Sunday
14 Dec 1915
Dear Mum

I have been bad about writing again but I had rather a job to get paper but I went into the nearest town and got this, its not nice but better than nothing. I arrived quite safely and have been given the best billet in the whole place, a room in a huge Chateau, with such nice people. The weather is absolutely hopeless. It has hardly stopped raining since I have been here and the aerodrome is one mass of mud and water and impossible to get out of with an observer and hard enough by yourself. I haven't been up yet on account of this, but I ought to get a fly tomorrow if it doesn't rain in the night, and it certainly doesn't look like raining now. We had a concert the other night and I sang Sister Susie with variations, very badly I'm afraid, but I think it amused the men. The next night we had a Cinema show got up by Major Blackburn, that is the person who used to be at Aldershot, do you remember? I went and saw his wife at Sandhurst. He is such a nice man, and wanted to be remembered to you. We are a long way back about 11 miles and can hardly hear the guns at all. There is an awfully nice lot of people here and jolly good mechanics which is something anyhow. Thank you so much for the letter, and I got the scarf and the shoes which you forwarded to me today. Such a lovely scarf, it ought to keep me warm. The men love your parcels and think the jerseys just *the* thing for the winter. I am afraid there are hundreds of things I want. Do you think you could go to Andre's where you got my coat and ask him to send me out the rest of that flying cap of his, it is a part which goes over the chin to keep it warm. Tell him I have got buckles for it on the cap. Do you know the kind of snowboots you have been sending out to the men, big ones which come right over your ankle. Do you think you could get me a pair of those if possible they are the only things which keep you warm when flying. I want *huge* ones about size 12. The man will probably tell you they are too big. Don't take any notice of him at all. I would also like an ordinary pair of *chamie* (I don't know how to spell it) gloves to go under my fur ones. Could you go to Weinburgs in Bond Street and ask him to send me out cigarettes regularly. I can get all the tobacco I want out here. I am afraid I have asked you to do an awful lot, and you are so busy. The coat is excellent and the envy of everyone. A Frenchman landed just outside our aerodrome today having lost his way. Such a funny little man about 2 foot high and legs like matches anyhow he seemed quite happy and jumped about with excitement when his engine wouldn't go. We got him off at last and he went off waving his hand. I enclose a cheque to cover expenses for all the things.
Heaps of love from
Ian

Flight contributed a descriptive article on the subject of clothing in November 1915. In the light of the preceding letter, articles of this sort must have been very valuable to the confused aviator in France.

In my quest on behalf of the aviatic world I have made up my mind to note only what I consider a real boon, and with that thought in my mind, naturally Harrod's suggests itself for a first visit . . .

Here are *some* of the lines I recommend for inspection. Long coats, short coats, three-quarter coats–how shall I ever describe them? Sheepskin jackets, lambswool waistcoats, leather suits, overalls, underalls, gloves, boots, caps–oh dear! A beautiful aviator's three-quarter coat (the adjective governs the coat) in black or tan sheepskin, chrome dressed, and really soft. All-round belt, large side pockets and diagonal map pocket; double breasted, with extra wide overlap fronts, and double collar to turn up, with cross piece to button over the throat. Lined with dark grey fleece, it makes a

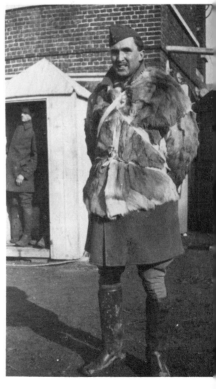

Personal improvisation in the early days of the war.

really serviceable coat. The same in half length, at less money but no reduction in quality.

Complete leather trouser suits in black or tan, and a naval coat, also in both colours, with the usual side pockets and large map pocket.

Gloves of every description, lined with every conceivable material calculated to keep the hands warm. One, in particular, I noticed, with the underside of the finger tips left unlined in order to facilitate the feeling of switches. Another good line is a gauntlet glove, lined with fleece, with waterproof canvas backs and leather fronts, and strap fastening.

Flying caps of every description, lined with fur, or fleece, or unlined. Helmets, wool under-caps. Long boots, short boots, boots lined and boots unlined; everything one could possibly want in the way of equipment . . .

The General Aeronautical Company known the world over as the 'GAC'. Obtainable here is everything connected with aviation, from an engine to a pair of goggles. In clothing, they specialise in kapok, that wonderfully light, waterproof, warm, vegetable wool which, in addition to other qualities, is buoyant in water, thus acting as a life-saving jacket should mishap befall an aviator when over water. The material is used in a number of forms, principally in the shape of undercoats and waistcoats. In the waistcoat form, they may be had made up in the ordinary way,

An RNAS pilot in a BE2c wearing a Warren helmet.

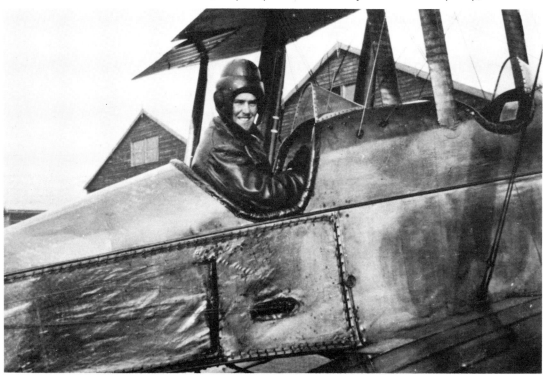

to button down the front, or simply with straps over the shoulders, looking very much after the style of the cork jackets worn by lifeboat men.

In jacket form, it is made not quite so thick, and with sleeves, the kapok in this case being sandwiched between flannel, and made more with the idea of warmth than with life saving, although even with the lesser amount of kapok, the buoyancy is remarkable, and quite capable of keeping the wearer afloat in smooth water.

A one-piece suit in black, chrome-dressed leather, is also a speciality, it being also kapok lined, although, of course, to a lesser extent than the life-vests primarily intended for life saving. Nevertheless it should be very buoyant, and it certainly is beautifully made. It has an all-round belt and the leg is fitted with buttons from some distance upwards from the ankle, so that the wind is prevented from entering . . .

And so to Burberry's in the Haymarket. To expatiate on Burberry goods is about on par with trying to paint the sky blue, but as the lines there dealt in are entirely

Burberry, we ask for Mr Doman, and proceed to investigate their unique examples of high-class tailoring.

The 'Tie Locken' long flying coat is just the very thing for the purpose. The material is absolutely weather-proof, and it has an exceedingly great overlap front, extending right to the bottom, so that the legs cannot get wet through the blowing up of the coat. Further to prevent this from happening, there are straps through which one can pass the legs, which yet do not interfere with walking. It is made in two colours, khaki for military wear, and blue for naval wear, and being of material in the place of the usual leather, it is almost impossible to tell the coats from those cut from ordinary cloth. The belt is of the all-round type, but, as usual, it adjusts both back and front. Side pockets are provided and the collar can be used in three positions. A feature of this coat is that there are no buttons – all fixing being accomplished by easily-adjusted straps and dome clips.

'Gabardine' is a material used in many ways, including the manufacture of complete flying suits, after the style of the well-known leather suits, but here with distinctive features with regard to cut and finish. The material is weather-proof, as distinct from water-proof only. It will throw off any quantity of rain, and yet give ventilation to the body, which it also keeps warm at low temperatures. Sir Ernest Shackleton used a suit of this material on his Antarctic Expedition, and expressed, in a letter, his admiration of its ability to keep out the wind and cold in a blizzard. As all the world knows, military coats and uniforms, as also naval, may here be obtained in the firm's weather-proof materials – these including those of the Royal Flying Corps.

In addition there are fur-lined under-jackets with sleeves. Long undercoats lined with camel fleece. Flying caps lined with fleece or gabardine, and warm clothing of every description.

One good line in gloves is a pair made of horseskin. To look at they appear to be brown suède, but their speciality is that they always remain soft. When wet they do not get 'soggy', and when they dry they dry soft and flexible, so unlike the usual leather glove, which will generally dry hard and stiff. They are, I need scarcely say, lined throughout with fleece.

And so on round the stores; to Gamages where the author sees a one-piece leather suit called a 'Blériot', the advantage of which is that it has no ends to flap around and get in the way, to Selfridges, to Dunhills of Conduit Street, who sell Japanese paper under-jackets, and finally to Robinson and Cleaver of Regent Street.

The airman had every opportunity to wrap himself up in layers of silk, wool and leather, and the more layers he had on the warmer he would be, but this meant that any physical manoeuvres on the part of the pilot or observer while in the air were carried out only with considerable difficulty. This was so with aerial photography, which became an accomplished art in World War I, for in cold conditions an observer had to operate his camera and change plates encumbered by gauntlets, bulky clothing and a roaring slipstream. The task of operating an offensive weapon was hampered by similar difficulties. By 1915 most aircraft had defensive armament, but many squadrons had been allocated a single-seat Scout or fighter in which a chosen few could ascend and endeavour to shoot down the enemy. To operate an offensive weapon, such as a Lewis gun mounted on the upper mainplane centre section, was extremely difficult. Louis Strange, a nineteen-year-old Lieutenant in No 6 Squadron, was involved in a frightening incident which occurred as he was attempting to change ammunition drums on just such a gun. At 8,000 ft while flying a Martinsyde single-seat aircraft allocated to No 6 Squadron, he was attacked by a German Aviatik. He fired a whole drum of ammunition at his adversary, then had to re-load. To do this he had to stand up in the cockpit and remove the empty drum. It stuck and his exertions caused him to lose his balance, releasing the control column held by his knees. The aircraft was very unstable and promptly inverted, with Strange gripping the empty drum. He dangled in space until, by some incredible feat of strength, he managed to swing himself back into the cockpit and right the machine. The violence of his efforts had thrown his seat out and broken all the instruments – a shaken and very lucky man returned. Safety harnesses were yet to be generally introduced.

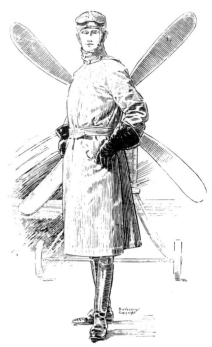

Skirts of The Burfron are shaped so as to shoot wet clear of the legs when seated. A great boon to the aviator, who thus escapes a wet seat.

New machines

The use of guns to attack the enemy in the air had the approval of many. As early as September 1914 No 4 Squadron, flying Maurice Farman biplanes, had Lewis guns fitted to the front nacelle. Because this was a pusher aircraft, with the propeller positioned behind the pilot, a clear field of fire could be enjoyed, although these machines lacked the speed to make any decisive attacks. The Vickers Gunbus, which came to France in 1915, also had a pusher configuration, but because it boasted a more aerodynamic outline it became a successful fighting aircraft. This supremacy lasted until the Fokker interrupter gear was introduced which allowed a machine-gun to be aimed and fired through the propeller arc of a tractor aircraft. Air fighting on the Western Front now began on a serious scale. With the interruptor mechanism mounted on a Fokker EIII monoplane, the tool of flying 'Aces' was available; the age of dog-fights and heroes had arrived. For four months the Fokker scourge rained death on Allied aircrews, until the spring of 1916 when the single-seater 'pusher' fighters, the DH2 and FE8 and two-seater FE2bs, were introduced.

A pilot of an FE2a wearing a long leath flying coat, a flotation waistcoat and speci non-flammable goggles produced by t London Label Company.

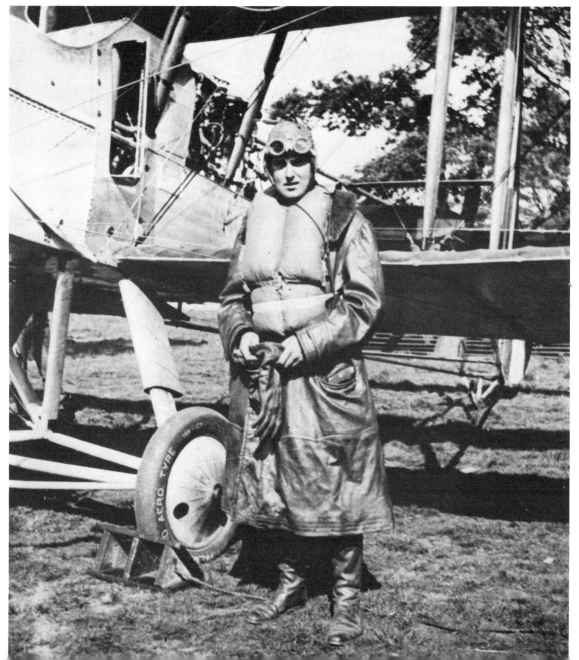

The FE2bs were pusher biplanes carrying a pilot and observer in tandem. A machine-gun in the front cockpit gave a good arc of unobstructed fire but subjected the observer to a full blast of slipstream, for these unfortunate observers had to stand up to be able to use the gun at all angles. Often with only his feet and ankles below the gunwale of his cockpit, the observer had to load and fire his guns while the pilot put the aircraft through all manner of evasive manoeuvres. He had to hang on to his guns or their mountings to stop himself from falling out as no harnesses were fitted. Frequently the observer would be saved from falling out, particularly when wounded, by the pilot's grabbing him.

The DH2 first entered service on the Western Front with No 24 Squadron, led by Major Hawker. Again a pusher design, but a single-seater, it had an excellent performance for its time and proved very successful. The chief drawback with this machine as with all 'pushers' was the appalling cold suffered by the pilot because there was no engine in front of him to keep him warm. This was fatally demonstrated by Second Lieutenant F. A. Archer, 'C' Flight Commander of No 24 Squadron. Lieutenant Archer's DH2 was seen to spin into the ground on 9 February 1916. It was the end of a long patrol, and it was generally held that his legs and arms became so numb with cold that he could not control the aircraft. He was killed.

A danger with the pusher designs was the dramatic aftermath of a forced landing. The heavy engine, particularly of the FEs, would move forward on impact and crush the pilot and observer in the nacelle. Often the only hope was that, on impact with the ground, the crew would be thrown clear of the aircraft. Unfortunately, special clothing could not mitigate this hazard. The French introduced a new fighter, the Nieuport, which was a tractor design and ten mph faster than the RFC machines. Its configuration was ideal, and with interrupted machine-guns it became an extremely desirable combat aircraft. The tractor design offered better weather protection to its pilots, some warmth from the engine and a better chance of survival in a crash.

In May 1916 the Sopwith 1½ Strutter aircraft appeared at the Front with No 70 Squadron; all these machines had synchronised machine-guns and could therefore act as bombers and fighters in the same formation. Later in the same month Captain Albert Ball, flying a Nieuport 16 Scout, shot down his fourth and fifth victims. Albert Ball, one of the great aces, hated any sort of encumbrance and flew without helmet or goggles in all weathers and aircraft. Ball was not the only person to fly without helmet or goggles, and to disregard the general rule that all exposed flesh must be covered, even if only with whale oil, to prevent frostbite. Also in May 1916, the County Chemical Company produced the 'Chemico' bullet-and-bayonet-resisting body shield. Made from strips of fabric two and a half inches wide, and overlapping until at any point forty thicknesses would be the average depth, this shield was worn in the form of a waistcoat. At 27s. 6d. for a single and 47s. 6d. for a double shield the price was favourable. There is as yet no evidence that this was worn, even though Sir Arthur Conan Doyle in 1917 publicly calculated that forty to seventy per cent of minor casualties in the war could have been averted by using this product.

The year 1916 was to see great strides in aircraft development and an increase in military activities. During the Battle of the Somme, observation aircraft were operating every 400 yds of the front lines, flying contact patrols for the infantry. Aircrews were frequently flying four patrols a day, often unshaven, wearing their pyjamas under a uniform and flying-coat, as well as keeping their bedroom-slippers on under their snow-boots. When the weather improved their flying times would regularly total eight hours a day. Offensive bomber attacks were made up to thirty miles behind the enemy lines. The bombers were now escorted by fighters, although later for added defence two out of every ten bombers were equipped with two Lewis guns, acting as gunships in formation.

Supremacy for either side in conflict was short-lived. The strong aerial armadas of the RFC were shaken by a new German squadron, JG2, commanded by Hauptmann Oswald Boelcke. This and subsequent squadrons were equipped with Halberstadt and Albatros fighters. With two synchronised machine-guns and a better speed and rate of climb, they were superior to their opposition. The RFC had 380 aircraft at the front, the Germans 330, but forty-five of these were the new fighters. In October 1916 the biggest air battle of the war was fought when twelve RFC bombers with fourteen escorts were attacked by thirty German aircraft.

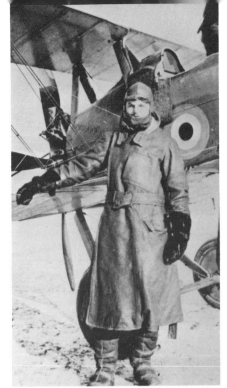

An unfortunate FE8 pilot.

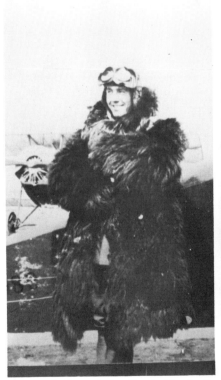

Roderic Dallas of the Royal Naval Air Service with his own solution to the problem of cold.

In September 1916 Flight-Sergeant J. T. B. McCudden shot down his first enemy aircraft. One RFC legend was about to start but, sadly, another ended, for on 23 November Major Hawker, VC was killed in his DH2, shot down near Bapaume by Richthofen. Not only was he a great pilot, but he would almost certainly have made a name for himself as an engineer. Together with warm boots he usually wore a leather flying overall, leather helmet, gauntlets, and a large sheepskin which covered his chest and shoulders and was tied around the waist, yet another example of the necessary personal improvisations if flying a DH2 was to be at all comfortable.

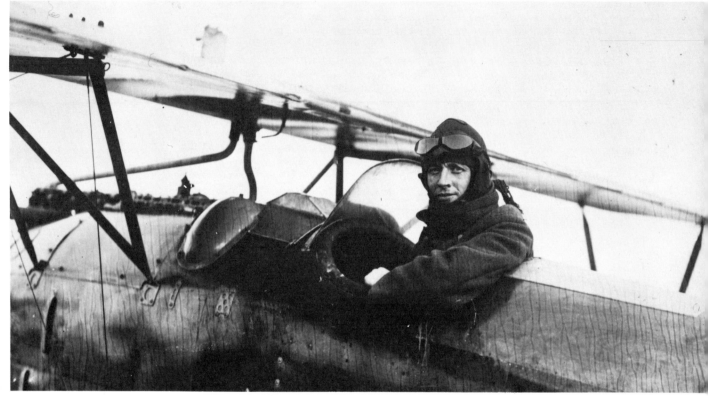

Scout pilot in an Albatros DIII.

Reinforcements to cope with increasing losses were obtained by switching squadrons around; No 8 RNAS Squadron found itself at the Front as a result. Moved from Dunkirk, the unit was equipped with Nieuports, Sopwith 1½ Strutters and the new Sopwith Pups. Sidney Cotton, an RNAS pilot who was a member of this Squadron, made a discovery which was to have profound effect on aircrews long after the First World War . . .

I always personally supervised the maintenance work on my plane, and one day in the middle of the very cold winter of 1916 I was tuning up my engine, dressed in dirty blue overalls, when we got an enemy approach warning. There were several 1½ Strutter fighters based at Ochey, and I took off with them and we searched the sky for an hour. We saw nothing and returned to the aerodrome. When we collected afterwards in the Mess everyone seemed to be frozen stiff. Everyone, that is, except me. One of the other pilots remarked on this, 'Cotton', he said, 'you don't seem to be cold at all. Why's that?' 'That's funny,' I said, 'I'm quite warm. And I didn't even have time to put my flying kit on! I was simply wearing my dirty overalls.'

I thought a lot about this, and I went to my room to puzzle it out. On examining my overalls I found they were thick with oil and grease, and I decided that they must have acted as an airtight bag and kept the body heat in. At this time, pilots in their open cockpits were suffering severely from the cold, and it seemed that I had a ready-made idea for a flying suit. Largely because I hated the thought of anyone else flying my plane, I hadn't taken leave since I went to France, but now I asked for leave and went to London, where I got Robinson and Cleaver to make up a flying suit to my design. The suit had a warm lining of thin fur, then a layer of airproof silk, then an outside layer of light Burberry material, the whole being made in one piece just like a set of overalls. The neck and cuffs had fur pieces inside to prevent the warm air from escaping. I had deep pockets fitted just below either knee so that pilots could reach down into them easily when sitting in the cockpit. I asked Robinson and Cleaver to register my design, and for a name I took the first three letters of my Christian and surnames – 'Sidcot'.

After twenty-one days' leave I returned to Ochey with several of the new flying suits, and I was able to report shortly afterwards to Robinson and Cleaver that the requirement had been fully met. I was the envy of the other pilots and several of them ordered their own suits from Robinson and Cleaver, who then tried to interest the RFC and RNAS in them officially. After searching tests the Sidcot suit later came into general use . . . Baron Richthofen, of the famous Richthofen Squadron, was wearing one when he was shot down.

The Sidcot suit has become perhaps the most famous clothing article associated with flying. According to the file AIR8/341 kept at the Public Records Office, it was invented and patented by a Mr J. J. Evans who was employed by Robinson and Cleaver, a friend of Sidney Cotton.

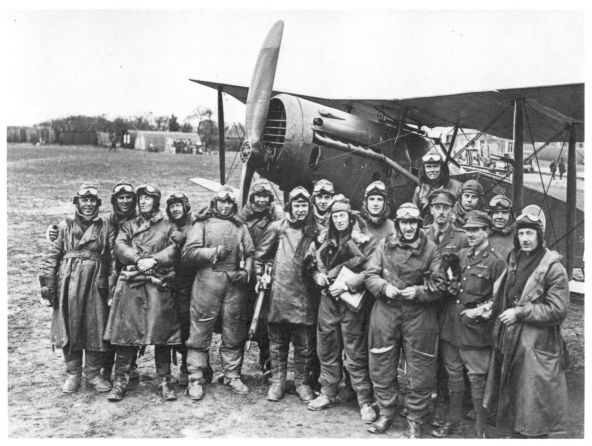

The Battle of the Somme ended in mud, snow and rain in November. A vast new expansion programme was planned for spring 1917, and German fighters were virtually outclassing every other machine, with the exception of the increasing number of Sopwith Pups. The German army had withdrawn to the Hindenburg Line and, as a direct result, reconnaissance flights increased in duration. Greater emphasis would be now placed on protection by formation; team work was reckoned to be the best way to stay alive. With very few exceptions even the great aces advocated such methods as being vital to the survival of airmen.

Crews of a Bristol Fighter Squadron showing the clothing worn by pilots and observers at this period of the war when Sidcot Suits were not generally available. 1st April 1918, the day the RAF was formed. Only three airmen are wearing Sidcot suits in the front row, the rest are wearing issue leather coats over 'fug' boots and their uniforms.

The average service of a pilot or observer in France was four months in two-seater and night-bombing squadrons, three and a half months in fighter reconnaissance and day bombers, and two and a half months in single-seat fighter squadrons. Calculations showed that during the Battle of the Somme average casualty rates were thirty per cent of the available aircrew. With the arrival of Boelcke and his new techniques and vastly superior Albatros DII fighters, the casualty figure rose to forty per cent. In April 1917 it rose to the fearful figure of sixty per cent, an average service expectancy of two months for all aircrew. The average number of flying hours for an officer at the Front, before he was killed or injured, was ninety-two. At this time a pilot was sent to France on active duty usually after only seventeen and a half hours' flying instruction. The experienced fighter pilots of the German Air Force lost no time in making 'kills' of these inexperienced young men in their outmoded machines.

Improvements had to be made, as supply could not keep pace indefinitely with demand. For obvious reasons it was decided to offer better instruction, and by September 1917 the instructional flying time per pupil had increased to forty-eight and a half hours. A School of Special Flying was established at Gosport, based on the fair assumption that instructors should be worthy of their pupils. It was inspired by Lieutenant-Colonel R. R. Smith-Barry, a veteran pilot who commanded No 60 Squadron in France. It was here that the classic training aid, the Gosport Tubes, was devised by Major Parker; a pair of tubes with mouthpieces at one end were fitted to the school's 504s and the other end was connected to rubber branch pipes leading to diaphragm earphones in the pupil's and instructor's helmets. By this means, and for the first time, a pupil could be verbally instructed in the air. This method of communication was cheap, needing no maintenance, and is still in use today in some aircraft, such as the Tiger Moth.

Problem of communications

Communication between two people in an aircaft had always been a problem, but with the introduction of the Gosport tubes, especially for instruction, the problem was to a large extent solved. There were, however, many other communications problems. From the beginning of the war it became abundantly clear that an observer in an aircraft must be able to communicate with an artillery post on the ground without having to land.

Observers of the Independent Air For collecting their weapons. Note the differe types of helmet, the Mk 1 goggles and the f boots worn over the Sidcot Suit for extr warmth.

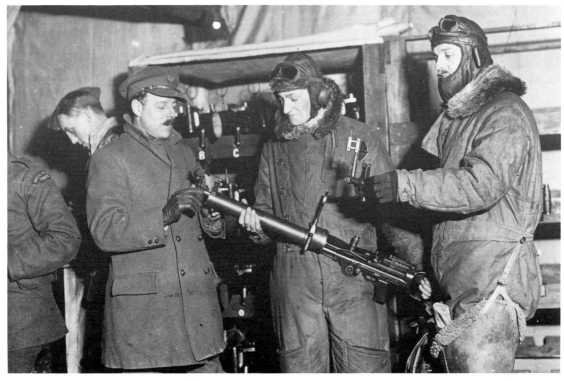

When the RFC first crossed the Channel in 1914 one aeroplane spark transmitter made by Marconi's Wireless Telegraph Company was supplied along with a carborundum crystal receiver. Helmets with earphones were issued to the few men in No 4 Squadron who were thus equipped. By 1918, 600 transmitter-equipped aircraft were available to help artillery batteries on the Western Front. Radio telephones were also being developed for air-to-air communications, and in July 1917 General Trenchard issued immediate instructions for ten transmitters and twenty receivers to be issued to equip a front-line squadron. In December, 200 helmets were ordered from Dunhills with fitted earphones and attachments for an oxygen-breathing mask fitted with a microphone. The mask was stiffened with whalebone to keep a good seal in a fierce slipstream. The microphone transmitter had to be easily detached from the outside of the mask. It was also possible to communicate by using a hand-held microphone.

During 1917 new advanced aeroplanes, such as the SE5, DH4, Bristol Fighter and Sopwith Triplane and Camel made their appearance at the Front. With more numerous and better-armed fighters, the truly awesome pattern of aerial warfare was at last formed. A striking example of this was recorded on the evening of 26 July 1917 over a small sector of the front lines: a number of German observation aircraft were patrolling at 5,000ft; at 8,000ft thirty Albatross DII fighters acting as escorts were in combat with seven DH5s; at 12,000ft ten Albatros DIIIs engaged thirty assorted RFC aircraft; while at 17,000ft ten more Albatros fighters fought with seven RNAS triplanes. Manoeuvrable, high-flying fighters were certainly now in evidence.

Concentration on clothing

Great efforts were made to improve the clothing situation, as aircraft were now staying airborne for greater lengths of time and were also flying at much higher altitudes than before. A report was issued in September 1917 which stated that five suits had been tested, including the Sidcot Flying Suit No 5 with RFC 'Maternity' jacket-front and pocket. Although this suit was not fireproof it was wind- and weatherproof, a fact gleaned from RNAS pilots who used the suit on flights up to 20,000ft. Obviously Sidney Cotton and his colleagues had proved the garment thoroughly. The report concluded that the Sidcot No 5 flying suit was regarded by all pilots as the most suitable and comfortable for flying.

Pilots of 54 Squadron, France, 1918, wearing standard RFC/ RAF clothing with the addition of a few personal improvisations such as scarves and gloves.

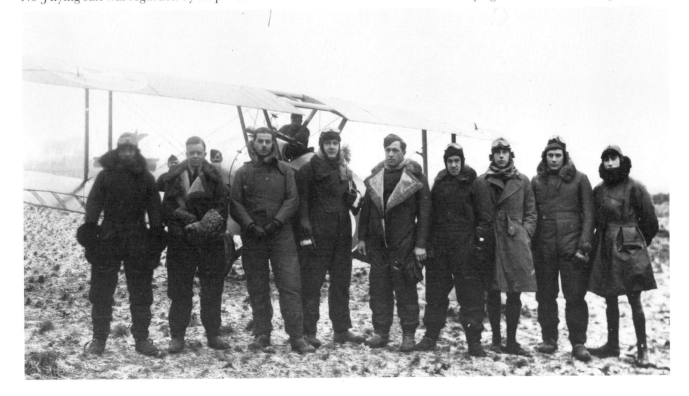

Robinson and Cleaver, the manufacturers of the Sidcot Suit, were expected to supply 200–250 suits per week fourteen days from the initial order. Deliveries were expected to increase to 1,000 per week, four weeks after the initial order. The RFC were anticipating a cold winter, so an immediate order was placed for 2,000 Sidcot No 5 suits, to sizes specified for the earlier leather coats they would supersede. By 28 November 1917, 1,126 suits had been sent to France, though only 371 were reported to have arrived. Requests were made for special shipping arrangements to improve the supply of these urgently needed suits.

By 18 December 1917, the order for 3,000 'No 55774 Jackets, Leather, Flying, RFC' was cancelled in favour of Sidcot suits. Instructions were given that the issue of leather coats should continue in Britain until existing stocks were exhausted. The Sidcot suits were to be sent first to the Expeditionary Force in France, then when more were available, to all units. In France a Sidcot suit was regarded as a very precious possession. When a new pilot joined a squadron he had to hand in his leather coat in return for the loan of a Sidcot suit. When transferring to another squadron, his Sidcot was re-possessed and his leather coat re-issued to him. By March 1918, 900 leather coats had been exchanged for Sidcot suits. All the squadrons in the 6th Brigade had been suitably equipped. Judging by the tremendous effort made to get it issued, the Sidcot No 5 suit was a really satisfactory answer to the airman's prayer. A testimony to its effectiveness was the growing pile of obsolete leather coats, so willingly discarded.

The RNAS had been making use of training facilities in Canada, and by April 1917 the RFC had established five trained reserve squadrons at Borden Camp in Canada (Nos 78 to 82 Squadrons). In April 1917 America entered the war. It was agreed that America would supply the RFC with 180 aircraft in return for experienced RFC officers to lead ten American squadrons. By the end of 1917 4,000 American recruits for the RFC were under training, and throughout 1918 200 pilots a month were sent from Canada to England. From a training manual we get some idea of the advice on clothing given to American pupils:

Plenty of clothing should be worn even in summertime. Leather overalls are the best for general work, and sometimes it is possible for a pupil to draw a flying kit on loan. This can be supplemented in wintertime by woollen sweaters, mufflers and helmets. The hands and feet are the parts of the body most likely to be affected by cold. Big boots are essential, and with a combination of silk and woollen socks or stockings, should help to keep the pilot warm. Goloshes or snow boots are also excellent, although somewhat clumsy. Many pilots object to the wearing of cumbersome gloves or boots, on the ground that it interferes with the touch and feel of a sensitive machine; but in the event of their hands or feet becoming frostbitten through insufficient protection, it may be remarked that they will have no feel at all. Fur gloves lined with wool are as warm as anything, and a fur flying cap, fitting close over the head, without ear holes, provides a suitable headgear and one on which it is possible to raise and lower goggles easily. Sometimes a pilot takes two pairs of goggles with him on a very long flight in case one pair should get lost, for it is a very bad thing to fly without goggles at any time. This is especially so on tractor machines lubricated with castor oil, which is most injurious to the eyes. The goggles should fit well and admit no draughts. Those fitted with Triplex glass are the best because, in the event of a smash, there is less chance of the glass breaking and cutting the pilot's face or eyes. It is a good plan to carry a rag to clean off the oil and dirt that collect on the goggles and windscreen from time to time, or the pilot may use the loose end of his muffler for this purpose. Newspapers provide an excellent protection against cold, and may be worn under the waistcoat or in trousers or boots. It goes without saying that damp footgear should be avoided at all costs, more particularly by those who are prone to chilblains and bad circulation.

Americans who flew with the French formed the Lafayette *Escadrille*. They used French aircraft such as the Spad and Nieuport fighters and dressed in French uniforms, wearing all manner of equipment. Edwin C. Parsons often flew in a loud-checked lumberjack's coat, worn over his uniform, crowned by a Roold crash helmet sporting a skull and crossbones painted on the front. Another famous pilot from this exclusive little group was Kiffin Rockwell who flew with a three-quarter-length sheepskin coat over his uniform. The wool was worn externally, making him look like a polar bear.

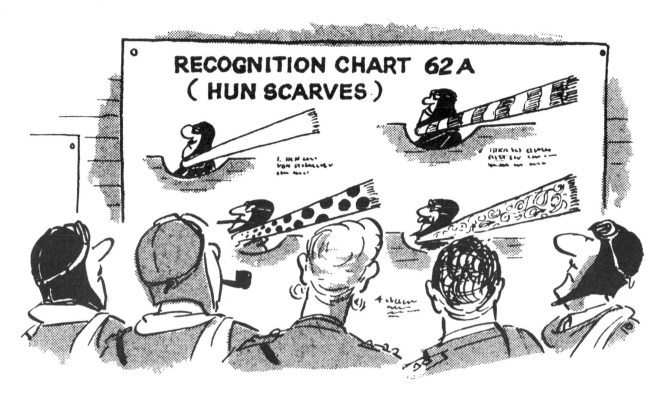

Most of the original members of the Lafayette *Escadrille* were killed during the war, although some were to command new American squadrons as they arrived in France. The sort of advice given to these men can be found in an article in *L'Aviateur* 1917–18:

> For long-distance flights one has to dress warmly, especially the extremities and, above all, the feet. It is quite easy to protect the hands by means of gloves and muffs fitted to the control column. However, the legs must remain free in order to have full control over the rudder. Therefore, as the weather gets cold or one finds oneself having to fly at high altitudes, one should put on warm trousers, boots a size too big and numerous pairs of socks (two or three), one of which should, if possible, be of paper. Thus it is necessary to forget all about high laced boots and thin socks; fur bootees are recommended for combating frostbite. Gloves should be large and not confine the fingers; flesh swells up when cold, and tight gloves can reduce circulation, allowing frostbite to set in. We would suggest, rather than gloves, however fur lined and warm, a pair of mittens with the thumbs separate: they are quite flexible enough and conserve heat much better.
>
> Under the helmet wear one or two balaclavas, one made of fine wool or silk (absolutely necessary). For facial protection, avoid grease at all costs; it freezes at low temperatures to a solid film which causes frostbite. If you wish, rub your face with glycerine and wipe it off carefully afterwards. The best way to protect the skin is to wear a leather or cloth face mask, fur lined, with an opening for breathing. Avoid mufflers, the long ends of which may catch in the struts, or even in the propeller. Never fly in a képi (service cap).
>
> Regarding the clothing of the body, a leather outfit is still the most practical. A good warm sweater and paper underclothing will enable you to face the cold comfortably. To avoid stomach chills, we recommend a flannel sash.

Towards the end of 1917, electrically heated clothing had been introduced by the RNAS for Active Service Units carrying out long patrols. Until this date warmth had been gained either by cocooning oneself in layers of clothing or by bravely resorting to the Edwardian 'winter-warmer'—a tin stuffed with smouldering rags—that frequently left nasty blisters. This equipment marked the beginning of technical developments in the realms of flying clothing. These suits would make life bearable for a few at least. Supply was on a fifty-per-cent-of-seating-capacity basis; hard luck on some. Each set of clothing issued consisted of an electrically heated waistcoat, a pair of gloves, and a pair of soles, plus electrical connections. The waistcoat was made of wash-leather, buttoning at the neck, with sleeves reaching down to the wrists. Two other circuits were connected through the waistcoat to the gloves, which were made of a cotton material, wind-proofed by a rubber coating and closed at the wrist by a light elastic wrist-grip. The gloves were made as thin as possible so as not to impair the touch. The other circuit was to the soles, worn inside flying boots next to the socks. The waistcoat was intended to be worn under the uniform tunic and flying coat. The gloves were also to be worn under ordinary flying gloves, although the latter would keep the wearer's hands warm on their own. A windmill generator mounted on the aircraft in its slipstream provided power for the heating elements. Although electrically heated clothing must have seemed to many to be a real luxury, it was by no means ideal. For example, often when a machine dived and the wind-driven generator produced too much electricity, finger burns became common. Extra body wrappings might restrict a pilot's movements but he considered them preferable to a heating apparatus which burned up or faded on him at the slip of a terminal.

Pilot and Observer of an FE2b night bomber January 1918, showing a wired waistcoat with electrically heated gloves. This would have been worn in conjunction with a uniform, "fug" boots and a leather coat. His colleague on the right is wearing a brand new Sidcot Suit. They both have the MK 1 mask goggles.

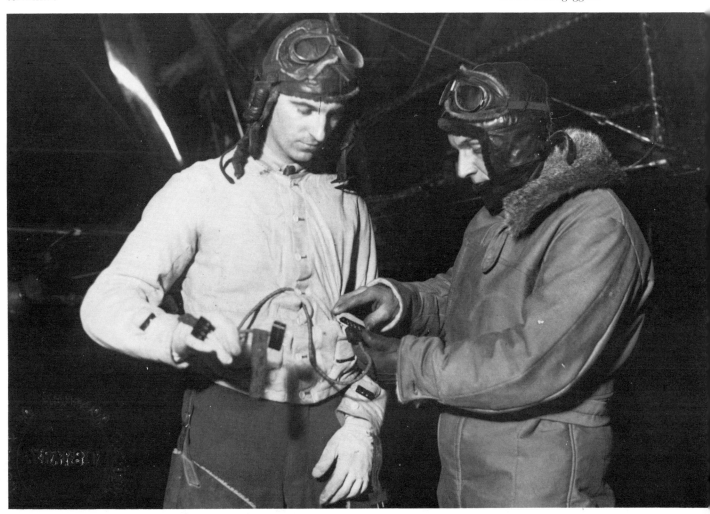

The French also had an electrically heated flying suit and it was this that became the model for the Americans. The French suit was an electrically wired overall. It was fur lined, and was much easier to put on than the RFC or RNAS types of waistcoat. It also had better insulation, so the wearer did not suffer from burns when elements shorted out. General Bolling, on 30 October 1917, sent a cablegram from his HQ in France stating, 'Each flyer sent to Europe should bring complete flying equipment. All clothing should be electrically heated. Sample satisfactory (French suit). Each flyer should have one piece fur-lined electrically heated equipment similar French type, shipped you, and type made by Revere Frères, New York.'

Colonel (later Brigadier General) William "Billy" Mitchell standing beside his Spad XVI, France 1918, in winter flying clothing.

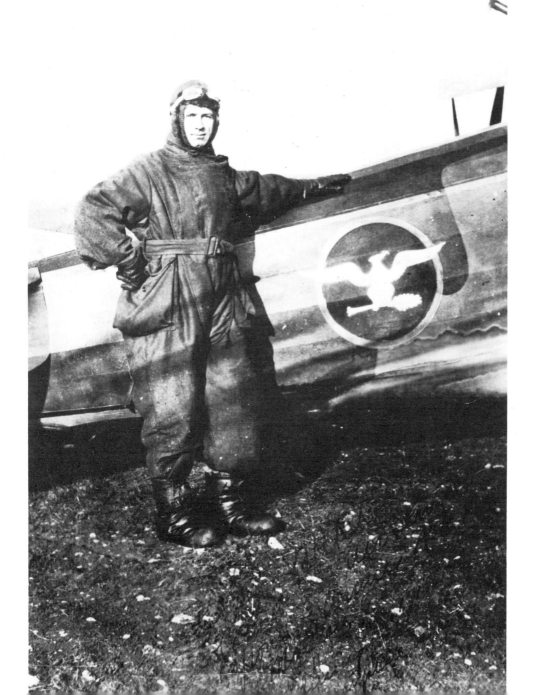

Despite this early request for good winter flying clothing, the matter did not receive special attention until 5 July 1918, when General Pershing cabled for 5,000 electrically heated suits. This order was placed with the Edison Electrical Appliance Company on 10 August 1918. The contract asked for 5,000 complete outfits comprising heated gloves, moccasins, helmets and a wired harness for suits. This order was not completed by the end of the war. Initially there was no means of controlling the temperature of the outfit, except by pulling out the plug in the event of overheating, but in September 1918 a test organised by the Edison Electrical Appliance Company was successful. Using a rheostat to regulate the temperature, the suit performed well for ten hours at an altitude of 17,000 ft in a temperature of −10°F. American airmen had to rely on silk scarves, fur-lined gloves and copious underwear to supplement the American Air Service flight suit, a one-piece overall that was waterproof and fur lined. On behalf of the Air Service 500,000 Nuchwang dog skins were contracted. This fur, called wolverine, had the property of repelling snow and ice; when brushed with the hand ice would fall off instead of matting in the hairs. Muskrat fur gauntlets and calf-length sheepskin moccasins were also supplied to American airmen.

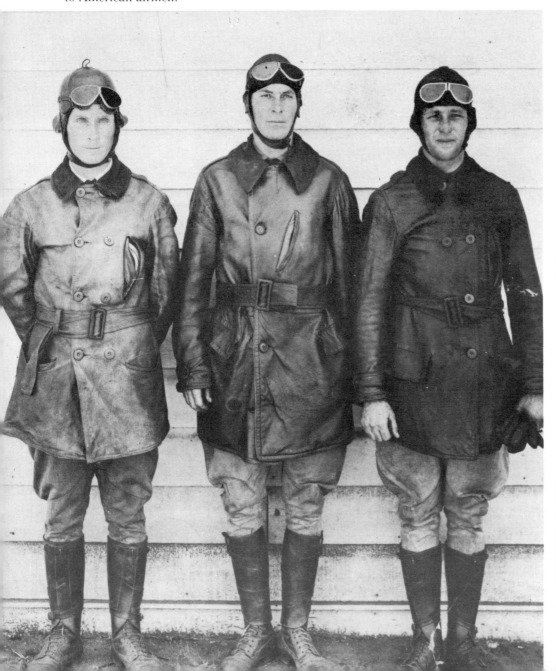

US Army aviators in standard flying clothin and Resistal goggles.

The crew of a German observation balloo appear to be wearing standard army uniform with the addition of a flying helmet an goggles.

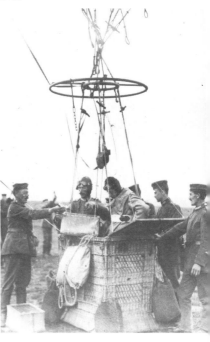

The Germans seem to have clothed themselves as opportunity dictated. Helmets of wool, cloth and leather were available. The standard issue helmet was made of shiny black leather, with a padded ring round the rim, and a single padded strip across the crown. Leather coats and overalls were also issued, many of which had fur collars. In summer, crews often just wore their uniforms with appropriate helmets, boots and gauntlets, supplemented with the service greatcoats. Among the more unusual items were infantry steel helmets and dark-lensed goggles. The Germans were great innovators and almost from the outbreak of war used electrically wired outfits in reconnaissance aeroplanes. From photographic evidence the equipment seems primitive, judging by the number of exposed wires visible even when the wearer was fully dressed. When clothing became scarce many pilots in the German air forces took to wearing clothing from captured RFC aircrews.

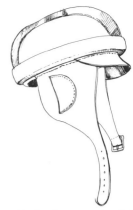

German Air Service protective flying helmet as issued during World War I. Made from black reinforced leather, with crash pads over and around the crown of the head.

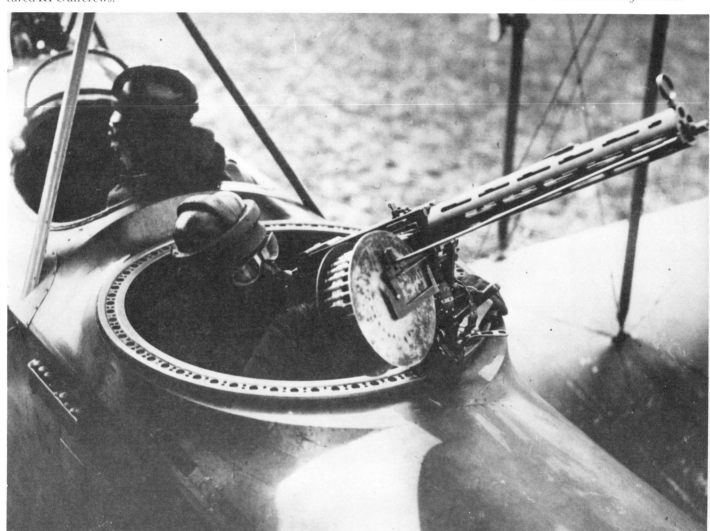

The German Air Force had, by 1918, adopted parachutes, and these no doubt helped save many lives. Observers in observation balloons had parachutes of the attached type, known as 'static-line parachutes', where the canopy was held in a container fixed to the balloon basket. When the observer jumped the 'chute was pulled from the pack. Zeppelins were equipped with similar devices, but these were discarded in 1918, because of the weight. The advantages of a parachute were obvious, and when the Germans equipped aircraft with the 'Heinicke' attached parachutes, pilots on our side of the lines became embittered when requests for a similar aid were refused on the grounds that they would only encourage airmen to abandon their aircraft unnecessarily.

German safety helmets.

Technology and the pilot

Germany also led the field in the use of oxygen by military aviators. When Zeppelins raided England in the early years of the war their crews had to resort to the use of oxygen, since heights of 17,000–18,000 ft were attained. Compressed gas was used in German airships until 1918 when the less bulky canisters of liquid oxygen were carried. At these altitudes temperatures could reach $-30°F$. Electrically heated suits were not worn in Zeppelins because of the weight penalties that the generating equipment produced. Fur-lined overalls stuffed with newspapers gave some comfort. Special helmets were produced for engineers who had to remain in the engine cars for long periods; these helmets were padded, with a glass visor at the front and rubber ear-pieces. Crewmen also wore specially constructed felt boots as boots with metal fitments were a fire hazard for men who had to pass along the narrow cat-walks, between hydrogen-filled gas-bags, in the hulls of the Zeppelins. Intelligence reports state that Zeppelin oxygen supplies were delivered to a simple celluloid mask which covered both the mouth and nose; a valve was fitted for draining condensation and another for expiration. The tendency for moisture to freeze and an unwillingness by crewmen to have their face covered led to the fitting of a pipe-stem mouthpiece, even these would freeze. In some cases a pilot flying at altitude would find that the pipe-stem had frozen to his lips and could be removed only at a lower, warmer altitude.

The soundproof helmet worn by Germa[n] airship engineers. It is equipped for use wi[th] oxygen at altitude.

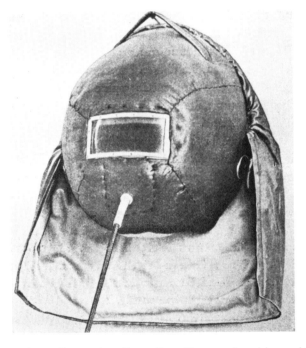
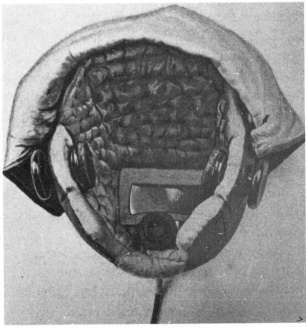

As well as using Zeppelins, German bombing raids were also carried out in twin-engined Gotha bombers, each with a crew of three. Armed with three machine-guns and 1,000-lb bombs, these aircraft had a range of 125 miles at 16,000 ft. The Gotha GIVs, flying from Belgian bases, were equipped with Ahrendt and Heylandt liquid-oxygen apparatus, with individual breathing tubes for each crewman. This apparatus was adopted by the US Army Air Service in 1923. Staaken R-VI machines were the largest aeroplanes to be used to bomb England, but as their bombing altitude was 15,000 ft, only a few of these aircraft carried oxygen equipment.

The first official British military oxygen equipment was produced by the Siebe-Gorman Company. This simple apparatus had a regulator valve with three manual settings, each increasing the oxygen delivery until a maximum altitude of 29,750 ft was attained. The oxygen came from one or two oxygen flasks, each containing 500 litres of gas. A rubber mask covered both the mouth and nose. Major George Dreyer, RAMC, devised an aneroid-controller regulator which was more efficient than the Siebe-Gorman type when it came to conserving the contents of the cylinders. The mask which accompanied this equipment was light and comfortable and eliminated frostbite. Manufacture of the Dreyer equipment started in April 1917 and approximately forty sets were in use with the RFC by December 1917. The Americans modified the Dreyer apparatus and had 200 units sent to France in May 1918. There is, however, no record of the equipment's having been used by the eight American DH4 Squadrons for whom they were intended.

The Observer of a DH4 having adjustments made to his oxygen equipment. February 1918.

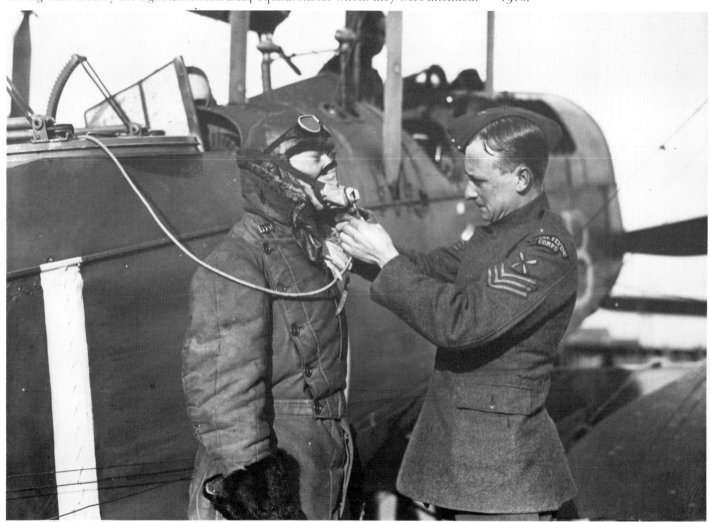

For some time it had been abundantly clear that the organisation of British air power was defective. The RNAS rarely came into contact with the enemy and had relatively little to do, whereas the RFC was unable to cope with its commitments. General Smuts of South Africa was asked to submit a report on the subject and proposed that a united air service be instituted under the control of an Air Ministry. On 1 April 1918 the Royal Air Force came into being. Shortly afterwards a long-range bomber force known as the Independent Air Force was established under the command of General Trenchard, a staunch protagonist of a policy of aggression. Equipped with DH4s, DH9s and Handley Page 0/400s they effectively bombed many targets in Germany. Of the men who flew these aircraft little is recorded so far as discomfort was concerned other than that they were equipped with rather inefficient electrically heated suits. By July 1918 2,171 electrically wired suits had been shipped to France; the waistcoats of these were made of Burberry material. The heated gloves often failed to work as the wiring broke with continual flexing. The foot heating was also unreliable as the electrically heated soles, made of mica, cracked with use.

Crews of bombers were also issued with oxygen equipment. In August 1918 the Air Board approved specifications for the Mk I detachable oxygen mask and flying cap with wireless equipment. The flying cap was close fitting, made of black chrome leather lined with nutria fur, with cap pockets for wireless telephone receivers; the weight was not to exceed one lb. The mask was made from black chrome leather also, and lined with waterproof fabric and nutria fur, and had an aluminium conical metal cap at its apex. Louvres were provided for the admission and exhalation of air. A small strip of lead was sewn into the top of the mask, so that it could easily bend round the wearer's nose, making a comparatively airtight joint. Elastic and mohair lacings made the whole helmet assembly a comfortable fit. The aircraft equipped were DH4 bombers, which were intended to fly on bombing raids at high altitudes over Germany, although heights of above 18,000 ft were still the exception. Oxygen equipment was primarily introduced for use by bomber crews but, in spite of its obvious advantages, only one fighter aircraft was thus equipped by the RFC. This was a Bristol Fighter of 88 Squadron. It would certainly have been of great benefit, as these aircraft were, by June 1918, carrying out patrols of two and a half hours at heights of up to 19,000 ft. It is possible that other fighters may have had oxygen equipment fitted, but no record exists.

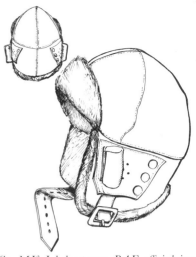

The MK I helmet was RAF official issue during World War I. It was made of chestnut brown chrome leather and fur lined throughout. These helmets retained the cylindrical leather pads in front of the ears seen in earlier designs. They were worn until the introduction of the 1930 Pattern helmet except in tropical climates, where the Type B helmet was worn.

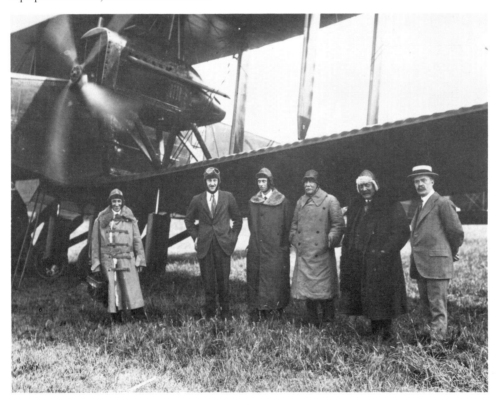

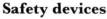

Members of the press in a motley selection of clothing about to be flown in a Handley Page 0/400 bomber of the Independent Air Force.

Safety devices

By late 1917, aircraft speeds at last exceeded 100 mph. Aircraft also became more manoeuvrable. With aircraft like the Camel some pilots chose to wear lightweight shoes or even carpet slippers to keep a sensitive touch on the rudder pedals. This was a problem that only personal improvisation could mitigate. The Sopwith Camel could respond so quickly to the controls that the pilot could be thrown out of his seat. For the first time aerobatic harnesses with shoulder-straps were fitted, rather than the straightforward lap belts as used earlier. It was not until late in 1918 that the Mk I observer's harness was officially recorded. This harness fitted the observer's body, over the shoulders, round the waist and under the crotch. Two straps attached to the waist joined between the observer's feet and were securely clipped at one point to the floor of the aircraft.

The ideal harness was devised by Oliver Sutton. It had separate pairs of straps with one pair passing over the pilot's shoulders and the other round the abdomen. Pinned together, these straps held the pilot securely in his seat, even when flying inverted. This type of harness could be quickly released, but would, under 'G' loadings, remain firm. A further advantage of a good harness lay in the fact that it prevented a pilot from being pitched forward into the instrument panel or guns in the event of a crash. In World War I little thought was given to 'G' forces. Many aeroplanes had severe structural deficiencies which limited their activities and often caused fatal accidents. In 1918 Garsaux began experiments with negative 'G' forces, using dogs in a centrifuge.

Test of buoyancy suits at the Isle of Grain, 1917. Laboratory tests for flying clothing were never as searching as practical demonstrations.

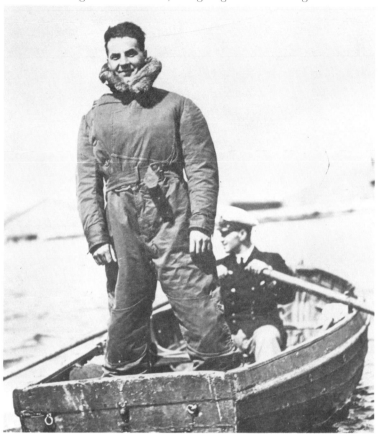

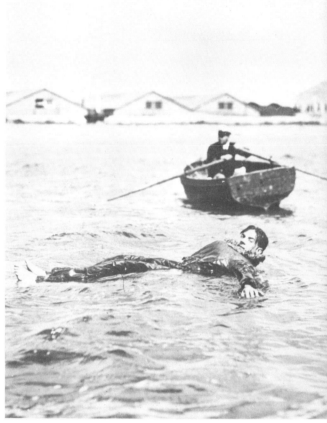

Another item of clothing that was not issued during the war but on which a considerable amount of research was carried out was an early form of immersion suit. In October 1917 RNAS aviators were acquainted with the Davidson life-saving dress, as worn by seaplane pilots. The wearer had to inflate the various flotation bags himself, but the suit was a great step forward in protection against exposure, the inevitable result of being immersed for any length of time. It is, in fact, unlikely that many survived a winter forced landing in the North Sea dressed in standard clothing. Tests were carried out with buoyancy suits at the Isle of Grain. The problem of survival in the sea led the RNAS to continue experimenting.

Although so much had been achieved by chance, genius and courage, so much still remained to be done. The problem of cold had in many ways been overcome but the cost was high. Oxygen and communications equipment, electrically heated clothing and safety harnesses were only slowly being introduced towards the end of the war. Parachutes had not been adopted by the Royal Air Force at all. In future, aircrews would be given every assistance; medical expertise would ensure this, but for the men who fought in the flying services during World War I this was only cold comfort.

Treatment of Government property

From the survivors of the greatest war mankind had yet engendered, a grateful Government lost no time in re-possessing its property.

Extract from Air Ministry Weekly Orders dated 5 December 1918:

1577—Return of Flying Kit on Demobilisation

1   All pilots and observers will be required to hand in their flying kit on demobilisation, and the value of any articles deficient or damaged by neglect will be charged against the individual responsible.

2   Pilots and observers of all ranks, serving at home or overseas, who have not yet been provided with FS Form 20 are forthwith to be issued with that form duly completed. If FS Form 20 is not available a MS certificate, signed by OC unit, detailing flying kit in possession of the individual concerned will be issued instead.

3   Pilots and observers no longer engaged on active flying, who have for that reason relinquished their flying kit, will be provided with a certificate to that effect signed by OC unit.

4   In the absence of documentary evidence (eg FS Form 20 or certificate) each pilot or observer will be deemed to have received a complete outfit, and will be charged with the value of any article not forthcoming.

5   A complete outfit consists of the following articles:

Boots, thigh or knee	pairs 1
Cap, fur-lined	1
Gauntlets	pairs 1
Gloves, silk	,, 1
Goggles, mask (without glasses)	,, 1
Glasses, triplex, tinted	,, 1
Glasses, triplex, non-tinted	,, 1
Suits, aviation; or jackets, leather	1
Overshoes, gaitered	pairs 1

6   This order will be repeated in the orders of all formations of the RAF, both at home and overseas.

7   The rates chargeable against individuals deficient of flying kit are as set out below:

	£	s	d	
Boots, thigh	3	18	0	pair
,, knee	2	18	4	,,
Caps, fur-lined (summer)		12	0	each
,, ,, (winter)	1	8	3	,,
Gauntlets, observer's, old pattern		17	0	pair
,, pilot's, old pattern	1	2	0	,,
,, pilots' and observers' (new pattern)		17	0	,,
,, linings, worsted		1	9	,,
Gloves, silk		9	6	,,
Goggles, mask, Mk I (without glasses)		12	0	,,
,, ,, Mk II (without glasses)		12	0	,,
Glasses, triplex, tinted		5	7	,,
,, ,, non-tinted		4	7	,,
Suits, aviation (Sidcot)	7	16	6	each
Jackets, leather	6	7	6	each
Overshoes, gaitered		9	10	pair

8   Adjustment of stoppages will be made as laid down in Weekly Order No 903 of 1918, as amended by Weekly Order No 1071 of 1918.

9   Full vocabulary rates set out above will be charged against all individuals deficient of flying kit on demobilisation.

10   It has been found necessary, for various reasons, that pilots and observers should carry out local alterations to articles of flying kit, particularly the conversion of thigh boots to knee boots, caps, winter pattern to summer pattern, shortening of leather jackets, etc. Articles so converted may be accepted into store without any charge against the individual concerned.

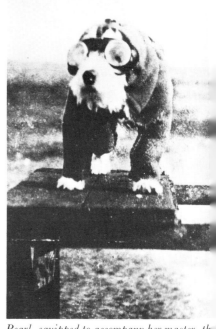

Pearl, equipped to accompany her master, the late Lord Grosvenor, into the skies.

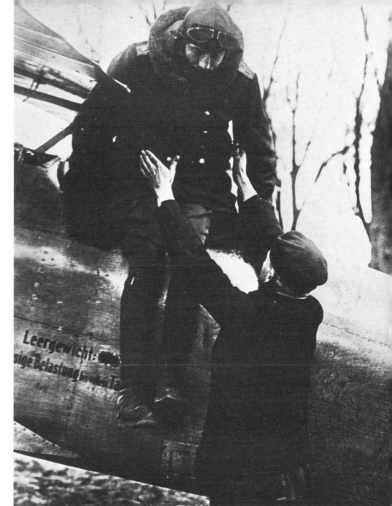

Richthofen being helped from Albatros.

Two British Artillery Officers preparing for an observation balloon ascent, May 1918. Note the different types of 'fug' boot, the variety of harnesses and the parachute packs in the background. Of all the British forces only balloonists were allowed parachutes.

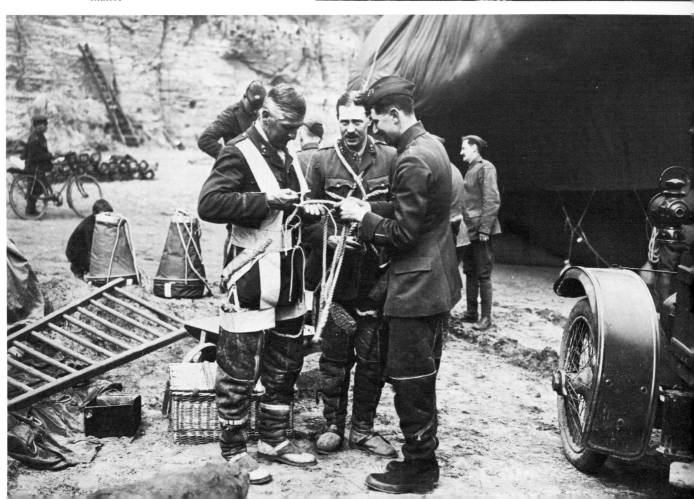

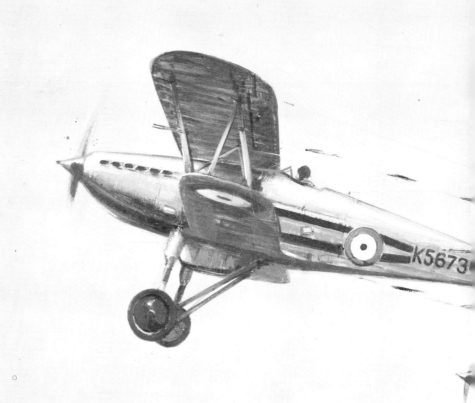

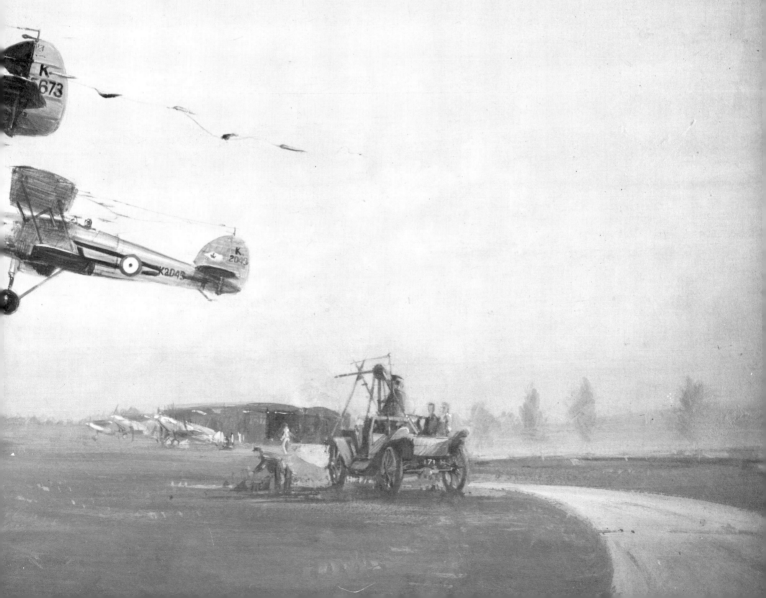

CHAPTER 3
HIGHER, FASTER AND FURTHER 1918–39

At the end of World War I thousands of aircraft were thrown on the scrapheap, tons of equipment buried in pits and large numbers of airmen demobbed. Only seven months after its inception the Royal Air Force was left to face the new peacetime era with a skeleton staff. Severe economic retrenchment and the antipathy of the Admiralty and War Office placed the RAF in a weak position, for the two senior Services saw the Air Force simply as a wartime expedient. As an independent Service they regarded it as anathema, since it had undoubtedly proved its worth in the war and this worth was a clear threat to their long-established powers. The Admiralty and War Office felt that the only sensible solution was to revert to the RFC and RNAS days when there were two Air Arms operating under the control of the Army and Navy respectively.

Fortunately the RAF was saved in its hour of crisis by the legendary figure of Major-General Sir Hugh Trenchard who was appointed Chief of the Air Staff. After many hours of battle round the conference table he succeeded in preserving the independence of the RAF, a position which, within a few years, it was able to justify. The RAF was now set to greet the peacetime era in its own right as an independent body. In 1918 when the Ottoman Empire collapsed, Britain had been given mandatory powers to assume responsibility for Iraq, Palestine and Jordan. On grounds of economy and in accordance with Trenchard's wishes the Government decided to use the Air Force to police these lands and quash any rebellions. The successful execution of these duties earned well-deserved recognition and respect for the Air Force. At home thorough training schemes were initiated at all levels, ensuring the provision of competent men for the Service. In 1920 the Central Flying School was established as a school for instructors, and the RAF Cadet College came into being at Cranwell; a few years later the School of Technical Training at Halton was founded.

The "Southern Cross" arrives at Croydon from Australia, July 1929. Charles Kingsford-Smith in his Sidcot Suit is second from the right.

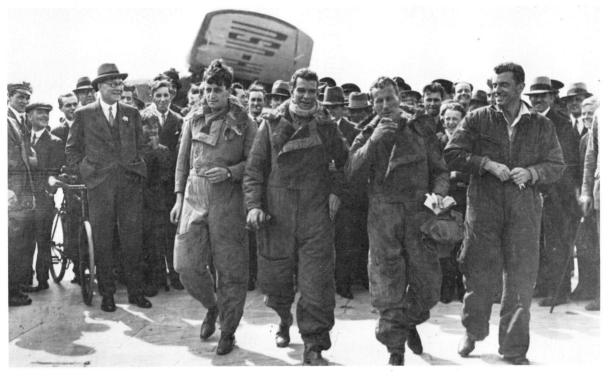

The inter-war years were years with a thirst for adventure, for record-breaking and exploration. These golden years of flying, nostalgic years for so many aviators, are associated with pioneering long-distance flights across and around the world, with attempts to break the world speed and height records, with the rise of commercial airlines, the widespread use of flying boats and airships, with the blossoming of the popular light aircraft movement and with the thrilling flying displays held all over the country. Names of national heroes such as Alcock and Brown, Lindbergh, Amy Johnson and Amelia Earhart immediately spring to mind.

In Britain progress in the aeronautical field in the inter-war period was achieved by the inspiration and efforts of a few. For example, it was almost entirely as a result of the outstanding generosity of a benefactress, Lady Houston, that the first flight over Everest and Britain's entries in the Schneider Trophy were made possible. The lean years of the twenties and thirties and resultant drastic defence cuts seriously curtailed any innovations that might have emanated from the Air Ministry. Biplane designs such as the Fairey Flycatcher, Gloster Grebe, Gamecock and Gladiator, the Vickers Virginia, Handley Page Heyford and the Hawker Hart and Fury epitomise service aircraft between the wars.

Monoplanes were being introduced in Germany in the early 1920s, but Britain failed to follow suit on any significant scale for another fifteen years, for the Fairey Battle, Bristol Blenheim, Armstrong Whitworth Whitley and Hawker Hurricane did not appear in RAF service until about 1937. For most of the inter-war years our defence forces were inadequately equipped with outmoded machines. Only the imminence of World War II and the rivalry of a country far advanced in the theory and practice of aeronautics would stir the conservative-minded Air Ministry to look actively and constructively to the future. It was not until 1936, three years after Hitler's rise to power and a year after the visit to Germany by two British Ministers, who returned alarmed by Germany's rate of re-armament, that a massive re-organisation and expansion of the RAF began.

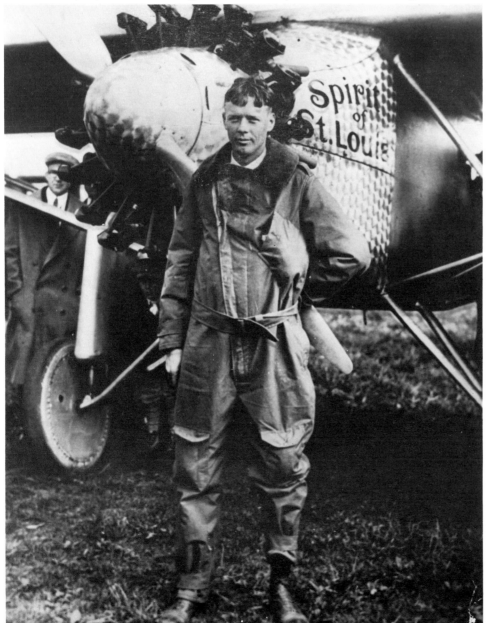

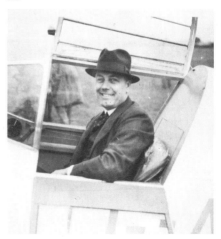

Lindbergh with the "Spirit of St Louis" after his successful solo flight across the Atlantic, 1927.

Edgar Percival in a Mew Gull of his design. He was noted for always flying with his hat on.

Spread of flying

The popularisation of private flying between the wars, the introduction of relatively cheap training aircraft such as the beloved de Havilland Gipsy Moth, and the mushrooming of flying clubs throughout the country opened up the world of flying to large numbers of enthusiasts. But since there was no radical change in aircraft design and performances for many years after 1918, there was no demand for any drastic change in flying clothing. The pilot sat in an open cockpit with nothing but a small windscreen to protect his face from the biting blast of the slipstream. Aircraft moved a little faster but the overriding problem was still that of protection from the miseries of cold and rain, and the answer still lay in cocooning oneself in as many layers of clothing as possible. For years after World War I civilian and military pilots alike continued to use wartime flying clothing, purchasing cheap war-surplus equipment that was so readily available from firms such as Lewis. The superb knee-length leather coats associated with wartime aviators became available as government surplus and adorned many a civilian pilot for years to come.

A display of ladies' flying suits at Harrods, 1928.

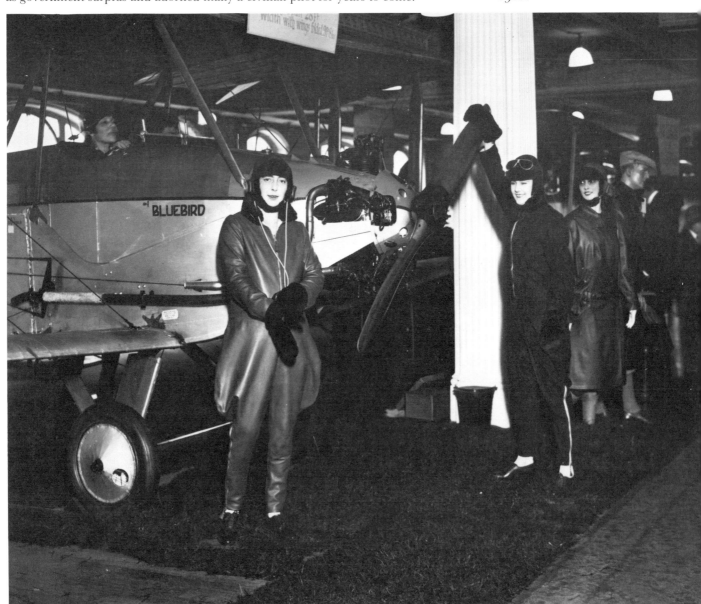

The more nonchalant of private pilots would be seen in a tweed suit in the twenties or maybe a cloth suit and trilby in the thirties, while those more concerned with the well-being of their suit rather than giving a debonair impression would envelop themselves in a pair of overalls or a Sidcot suit. Certainly the aviation clothing industry lost no time in gearing its designs to the image-conscious private pilot and as a result expanded rapidly at that time.

Even if, for one reason or another, you were unable to learn to fly you could always pay for a ten-minute flip to get the feel of the new dimension of flight. Many ex-wartime pilots earned considerable sums of money by giving joy-rides to local enthusiasts, and many distinguished aviators of later years owed their initial enthusiasm for flight to a brief joy-ride when a child. Barnstorming was a form of entertainment in the air, involving an aerobatic display, in the hopes of encouraging the spectators to indulge in a joy-ride. More often than not barnstorming was an informal yet controlled affair, but now and again a pilot's natural exuberance or plain stupidity would turn him into a dare-devil stuntman, enthralling and terrifying local inhabitants by performing breath-taking feats of aerobatics at low level. When the law began to clamp down on this wild sport, well-organised flying circuses began to appear, such as that run by Alan Cobham, and flying displays were placed on a more formal footing.

The bizarre craze of barnstorming is so often associated with America, but it had its own quieter parallel in Britain. Out to attract a following many of these exhibition pilots would dress in dashing attire to attract the ladies or, having sewn fraudulent badges onto their flying overalls, even claim to be wartime veterans. But perhaps more closely associated with the years between the wars are the magnificent annual flying pageants or displays held by the RAF from 1920, and by the SBAC from 1932, on Hendon Aerodrome, where many thousands of spectators came to watch new aircraft types being put through their paces.

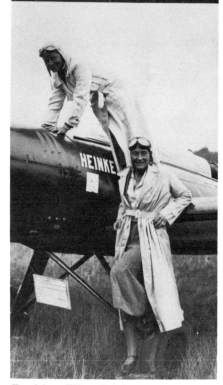

Fräulein Elly Beinhorn and Fräulein Mirow-Seelemann at an international air reunion at Heston, 1932.

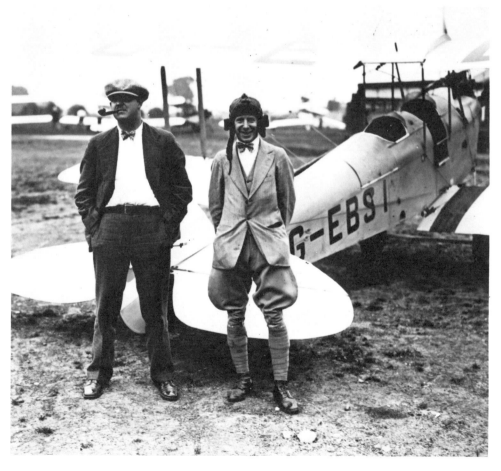

Inter-war optimism. Captain O. A. Gibbons from Canada and Donald A. Burpee from California plan to fly from Britain to California, 1927.

Miss Pauline Gower at the opening of Reading Aero Club, 1931. She is wearing Luxor goggles and has Gosport Tubes attached to her helmet.

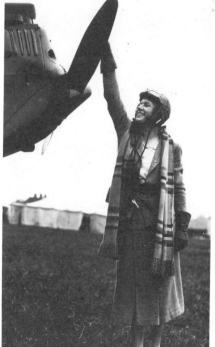

The Sidcot suit

As with civilian aviators, the standard issue, everyday flying clothing as worn by RAF aircrew during the inter-war years changed very slowly from that worn during World War I. RAF airmen clung tenaciously to their faithful leather jacket or coat. Leather jackets and trousers were issued by the RAF until 1922, and until the mid-1920s airmen were permitted to wear them instead of the standard Sidcot suit. The Sidcot suit, so longed for by pilots towards the end of the war, became the trademark of the military aviator long after the war had ended, and the thigh-length sheepskin boots or fug-boots which had effectively kept draughts out from under leather coats became obsolescent, since with the Sidcot suit there was no longer any need for protecting the leg much above the ankle. Knee-length boots were more than adequate.

The crew of a Handley Page V/1500 four engined bomber in their Sidcot Suits. They are wearing both the MK 1 goggles and special non-flammable goggles. 1918.

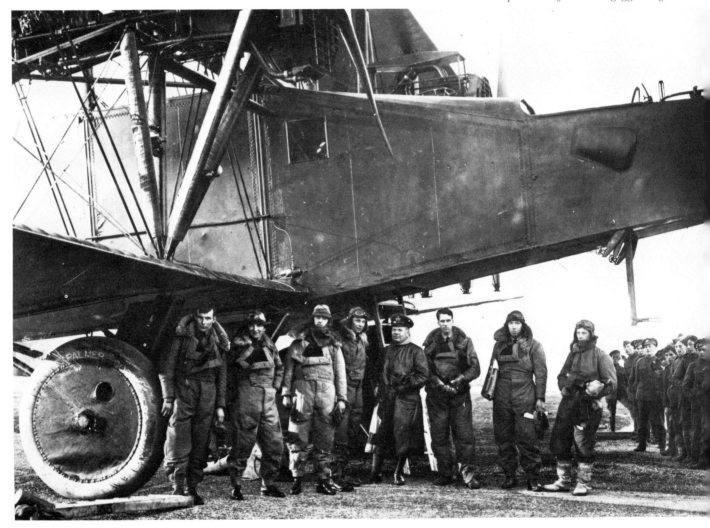

The all-in-one Sidcot suit, so popular when introduced towards the end of the war, was only in its infancy, and many modified forms of it were available throughout the inter-war period and World War II. By 1920 the suits were being fireproofed, a reassuring precaution against a hazard that all pilots dreaded. The RAF 1930-pattern flying suit was an all-in-one rubberised linen suit of a grey/green colour based on the Sidcot design. It sported a detachable fur collar and a large pocket on each knee and was done up by zip fasteners – a new invention. The suit was designed for wear with the wool inner ('Teddy Bear' inner) or the 1930-pattern kapok-quilted lining, but it was unpopular because it lacked adequate ventilation. It was superseded by the 1940-pattern suit.

The seven layers of a Sidcot suit, fur-lined boots, gloves and helmet were more than welcome on a chilly day, especially at any great altitude. Layers of underclothes and the odd woollen scarf were also of assistance. Extra-long scarves were popular for winding round the neck and then criss-crossing diagonally over the pilot's jacket or coat and knotting behind his back to prevent the jacket from billowing out like a sail when in flight. Loose scarves could, however, be extremely dangerous, and even the end of a tie which might flip up in the face at a critical moment could be disconcerting to the pilot.

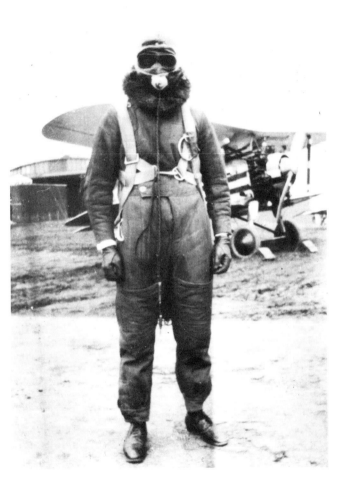

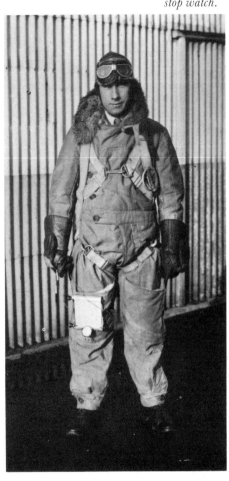

A pilot relies on good clear vision at all times. The continuous blast of the slipstream in an open-cockpit aircraft soon causes watering eyes, and the slightest speck of grit or dust can cause momentary blindness. Goggles have not only to protect the eyes but must also be designed so as not to restrict one's vision in any way. They consist of two separate eyepieces hinge-mounted on a frame at the sides of which are panels permitting ventilation; this prevents the goggles from fogging up. The Mks I and II mask-goggles were available with tinted or non-tinted Triplex glasses and were issued until well into the 1930s. By the mid 1930s the Mk IIIA goggles had been introduced. They had squarer lenses than their predecessors and were not fur lined. In 1923 goggles were issued with lenses of three different grades of density to represent full moonlight, half moonlight, and dark nights. These were intended to be used when practising night flying during daylight hours. In 1927 goggles were available with corrective lenses for airmen with defective vision. Many a near-calamity occurred when a pilot pulled his goggles out of his pocket, put them on as he opened the throttle and suddenly was almost blinded by an agonising pain. He had failed to check the cleanliness of the goggles and had been keeping them in the same pocket as his tobacco pouch. Tobacco dust had crept inside the frames of the goggles only to be dislodged by the airflow.

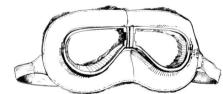

The price of progress

A pilot relies also on the sensitive and efficient functioning of his hands and feet, but these extremities tend to get colder much more quickly than any other part of the body. At all costs they must be kept warm and be prevented from going numb with cold. The more layers worn between which to trap warm air the better, and these layers must be loose rather than tight fitting. However, the more layers one wears the less sensitive is one's touch. It was quite normal to wear a pair of thin socks, a pair of thick socks and fleece-lined flying boots. Sergeant-pilots of the inter-war period were required to wear the heavy black leather service-issue ankle boots. This cumbersome form of footwear was not only insensitive to the controls but also extremely easy to put through the fabric skin of an aircraft wing. It was most important that a pilot did not get his feet wet when walking out to the aircraft, for any damp increases the risk of frostbite and makes that particular part of the body cold and uncomfortable. These factors resulted in the introduction, in 1930, of a knee-length, sheepskin-lined, light-brown suède boot with a rubberised section covering the foot. Six years later a black leather sheepskin-lined boot was issued. On his hands an aviator would wear a thin pair of silk inner-gloves which effectively retained the heat and were flexible enough to wear for operating the controls, and on top of these a pair of worsted-lined leather gauntlets, very similar in design to those worn by motor-cyclists and motorists of the pre-1914 era. One design had a flap-over mitten top which covered four fingers and provided extra protection against the cold. When not in use it could be press-studded back onto the glove, but it had the drawback of becoming easily detached and it tended to catch on switches. One trainee inter-war pilot landed nose-down in a ploughed field after his mitten caught the magneto-switch just after take-off. The 1933-pattern leather gauntlet did not have the extra mitten top, was elasticated round the wrist and had a vertical zip-fastener from the bottom of the gauntlet to the wrist on the palm side of the glove. By this date zip-fasteners were becoming a standard accessory.

Even a Sidcot suit sometimes failed to maintain a protective barrier against the ever-menacing cold. On bitterly cold days one's only hope was to put on electrically heated clothing – waistcoats, gloves and soles had been available in Britain since 1917, and were used by Brown when he and Alcock flew the Atlantic two years later. The Americans had developed an all-in-one electrically heated suit which they issued towards the end of the war but these early developments were not seriously continued until 1940. Although this type of clothing was a great comfort when working well, there were many times when the electrical supply would fail altogether or else develop a short-circuit, overheat and burn the unfortunate aviator. The lack of sufficiently flexible heating elements and of adequate insulation, as well as the inability of the aircraft to carry the added weight of a proper electrical system, resulted in the very slow development of electrically heated clothing during the twenties and thirties. The Royal Aircraft Establishment at Farn-borough produced an electrically heated suit in the late 1920s, and many were tested at Martlesham Heath in the early thirties, but progress was slow and suits were issued only to the lucky bomber or reconnaissance crews. A kapok-quilted lining was introduced in 1930 for use over an electrically heated lining to provide thermal insulation, but was extremely dangerous if worn without protective clothing on top since the kapok absorbed petrol easily and provided no protection at all if the aircraft crashed in flames. Martlesham even tested early cockpit-heating equipment, which proved ineffective unless tested at a low altitude on a warm day. When flying at high altitudes the cold was so appalling that in 1938 thermally insulated, brown leather jackets and trousers were issued 'for high-altitude flying where cockpit heating was inadequate'. Nobody defined 'inadequate', however, and the Air Ministry carefully regulated their issue. These suits were the prototype of the legendary Irvin suits of World War II.

America had done much research into Service flying clothing that was warm and yet light to wear. Fabric suits had been lined with fur or blanket material. The former proved too heavy and cumbersome, whereas the latter was not sufficiently warm. Reindeer-skin suits had been turned down in 1934 on the grounds that they were smelly and the skin shed its hairs. The final solution came in 1935 when Shearling suits made of lambs' pelts

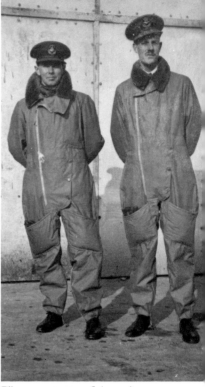

The 1930 pattern flying suit.

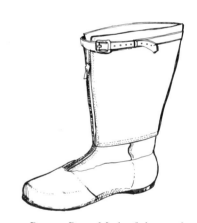

1930 Pattern Boot. Made of chestnut brown suede and sheepskin lined, these boots have rubber covered shoe section. The strap at the top goes right round the calf.

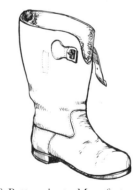

1936 Pattern boot. Manufactured in large quantities and officially superseded in 1940. It was made of polished black leather with sheepskin lining.

were issued. Designated Trousers Type A-3 and Jacket Type B-3 they were not dissimilar to the British thermally insulated suit of 1938. The Shearling suits were, however, unpopular because, although they were wind-proof and warm, they were bulky, heavy and inflexible and did not permit the escape of perspiration. In 1939 it was recommended that an intermediate weight Shearling suit should be introduced.

Crew of a Boeing B-17A wearing the first Shearling Suit, the A-3 Trousers and B-3 Jacket, 1939.

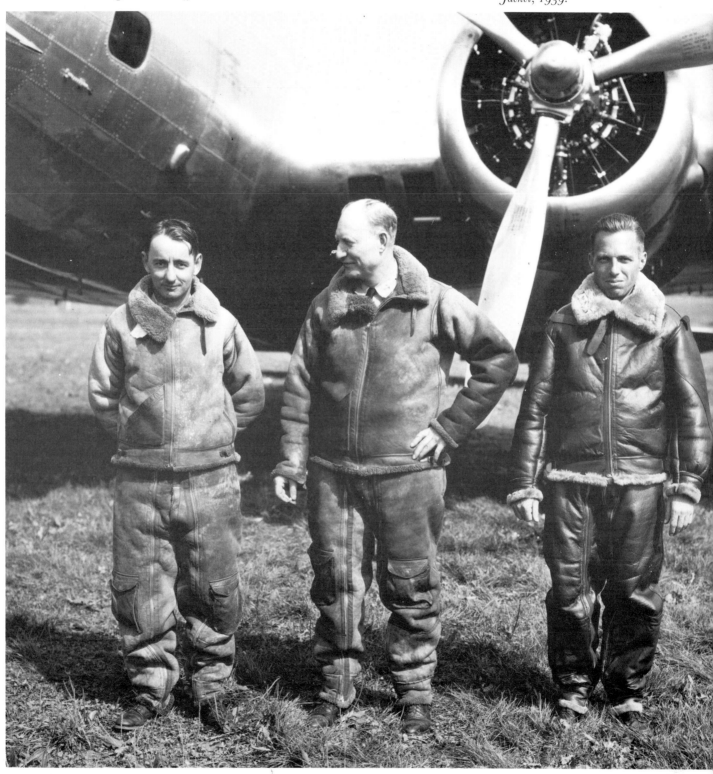

But England was not always shivering under dense layers of cloud, and it was the balmy summer days that saw the introduction of the inter-war pilot's distinctive trademark, the white cotton overalls. Racing motorists had made use of these white overalls for some years, for they were cheap, easy to fit over a suit to keep the latter protected from splattering dirt and oil, and of neat appearance when clean. Blue and brown overalls had long been worn by aircraft mechanics, but white overalls became the vogue for pilots, both Air Force and civilian, for use on special occasions. White overalls first became *de rigueur* in the RAF for flying wear as a result of their purchase by Auxiliary Air Force pilots, who were noted for being financially well off. These pilots bought their own flying kit and, as their trademark, adopted white overalls which they usually bought from Gieves of Bond Street. In order to save face, the regular RAF adopted these overalls for wear at displays. From the early thirties white overalls were invariably to be seen at the famous inter-war Air Force pageants and displays held at Hendon, and at innumerable air displays throughout the country. In 1935 they were officially issued to participants in the Mildenhall Review, with the squadron badge sewn onto the pocket. Even in winter months the white overalls were used in aircraft with enclosed cockpits.

American airmen, Captain A. W. Stevens and Lt. J. F. Phillips wearing oxygen equipment and winter flying clothing used on their photographic flights in Maine, 1932.

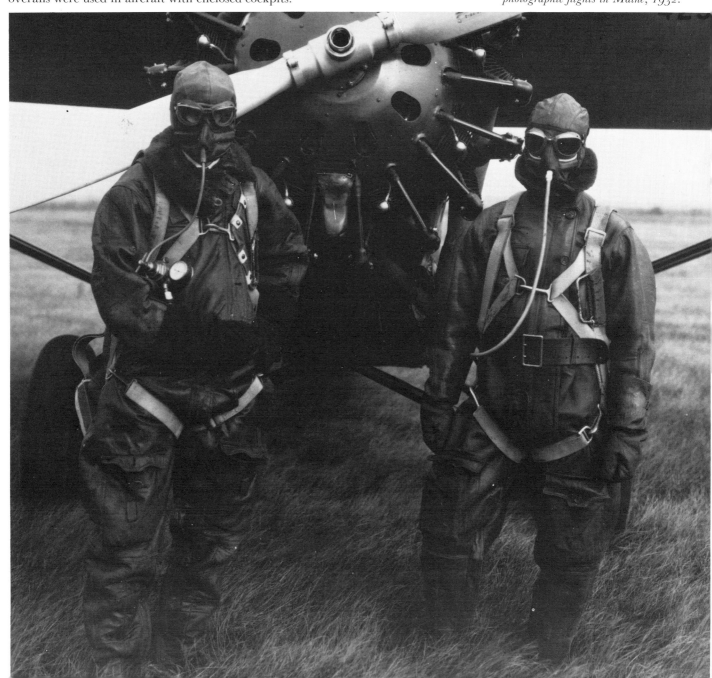

On the rare occasions when heat waves arrived in Britain, Service pilots would invariably ignore official clothing requirements and ascend in shirt sleeves, often choosing to leave helmet and goggles behind. The lack of goggles could be particularly dangerous, as impact at 150mph with a bumble-bee could blind a pilot, and hay, straw and dust were similarly hazardous. It was argued that this lack of protective clothing was not only more comfortable on hot days but also helped blow away any lingering hangovers. An added bonus came the airman's way in 1924 when 'drawers, cotton, long' were introduced for summertime wear as a welcome alternative to 'drawers, woollen'.

Flying on a warm summer's day in England was one thing, but flying on a hot day in the North-West Frontier of India or in Iraq was a very different matter. The RAF's strong commitments in the Middle East and India during the inter-war years meant that most people who served in the RAF between the wars had at least one spell abroad. With the sun beating down all day most airmen chose to wear the light khaki shorts which extended to the knees, although not long after issue they were usually chopped into short shorts, being more comfortable and cooler to wear. Shoes, knee-length socks, a shirt and a Wolseley helmet were also standard issue. Wing Commander Roderic Hill recalls the flying clothing worn in Iraq in the early twenties in his book *The Baghdad Air Mail*. In summer the pilots usually flew in a flannel shirt open at the neck, over which a spine pad was worn. This was a strip of thick material which buttoned on to the back of the shirt and which was sometimes lined with red to blank off injurious sunrays.

I was flying in my shirt and I wound my handkerchief round my neck to protect it from the sun. I had had a larger peak made to my flying topee by the tailor, but it was too flabby and blew up. What I do remember is the pitiless sun burning, burning down with an intolerable stare. And my shoulder, which was not covered by my spine pad, felt all stiff and bruised where the rays of the sun had fallen on it. I felt pretty worn out and tired, but still plugged on.

Auxiliary Air Force pilots in their distinctive white overalls.

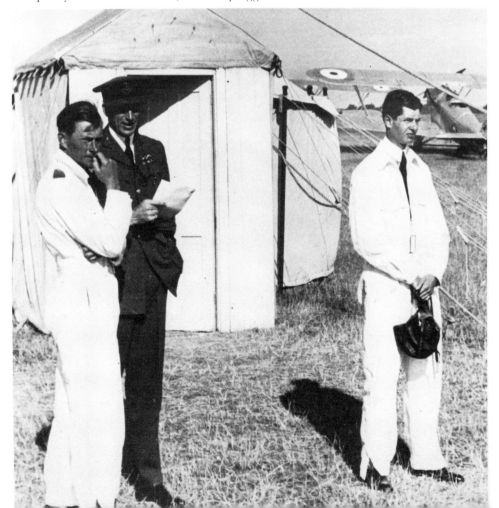

The Type-A cork aviation helmet was used in the years between the wars by aircrew stationed east of Malta. It had a smaller brim than the contemporary Wolseley helmet and was not unlike the pith hat or Baghdad bowler introduced in 1938. Because it was designed to be worn in flight it had two khaki earflaps which extended into a chin-strap to keep the helmet in position. In 1934 a tropical combination suit made of khaki drill was introduced. This one-piece 'romper suit', combining shorts and a short-sleeved shirt in one garment, owed its popularity to its comfort and relative coolness.

Flying in these hot parts of the world imposed many hardships on the pilot and his crew. When on the ground the men would sit around in shorts and a shirt that within minutes would be soaked with sweat. They had to wear gloves in the aircraft since the metal was far too hot to touch. But on climbing to any altitude they soon started to shiver with cold from the sopping garments. As a result many an airman suffered from bad head colds and chills.

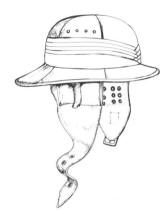

The Type A flying helmet as issued to aircrew east of Malta.

American flying clothing of the early 1930's.

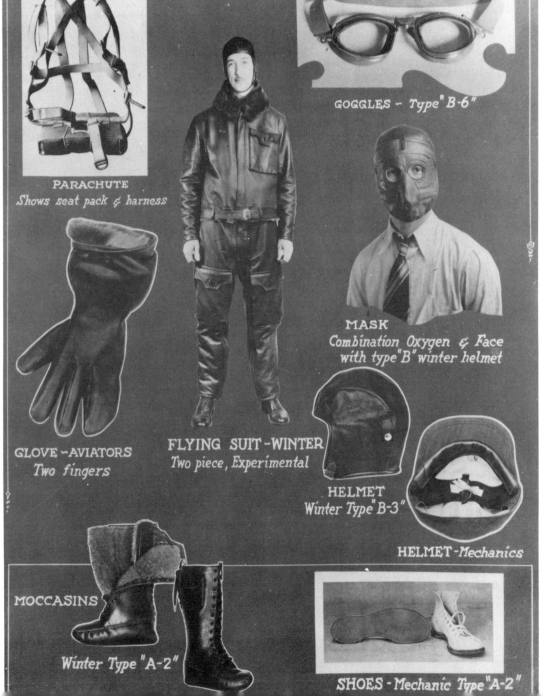

PARACHUTE
Shows seat pack & harness

GOGGLES – Type "B-6"

MASK
Combination Oxygen & Face with type "B" winter helmet

GLOVE – AVIATORS
Two fingers

FLYING SUIT – WINTER
Two piece, Experimental

HELMET
Winter Type "B-3"

HELMET – Mechanics

MOCCASINS

Winter Type "A-2"

SHOES – Mechanic Type "A-2"

Developments in communications

Communication between pilot and observer or instructor and pupil had always been a difficult task above the roar of the engine. Shouting was not very effective as one soon became hoarse; notes were sometimes frantically scribbled, special hand signals used, or for teaching purposes the instructor would exaggerate the movement of the controls to attempt to put a point across. It was undoubtedly a great boon when Gosport tubes were introduced towards the end of the first war. The equipment consisted of two six-foot lengths of flexible tubing together with a pair of earpieces and mouthpiece for pilot and passenger. Even today they are widely used by the vintage aircraft pilot. During the inter-war years Gosport tubes became a vital piece of communications equipment for aviators, especially those under instruction, and flying helmets were originally adapted, and later designed, so that the earpieces could be incorporated. The 1930-pattern flying helmet was made of a chestnut-coloured chrome leather, unlike the later helmets which were more the colour of dark peat. It was lined with chamois leather, was elasticised at the back of the neck and had ear-pads and leather flaps fastened by press-studs to hold the earpieces of the Gosport tubes in position. White twill flying helmets were frequently worn in the inter-war period – again fitted for Gosport tubes. Many of these tubes were issued in 1920 to flying training units for use in Avro, Bristol Fighter, DH9A and Short 184 machines.

Captain of an Imperial Airways Handley Page 42 wearing the newly introduced smart uniform and a Marconi anti-noise flying helmet designed to minimise extraneous noise thus allowing better R/T communication. This helmet first appeared in 1927.

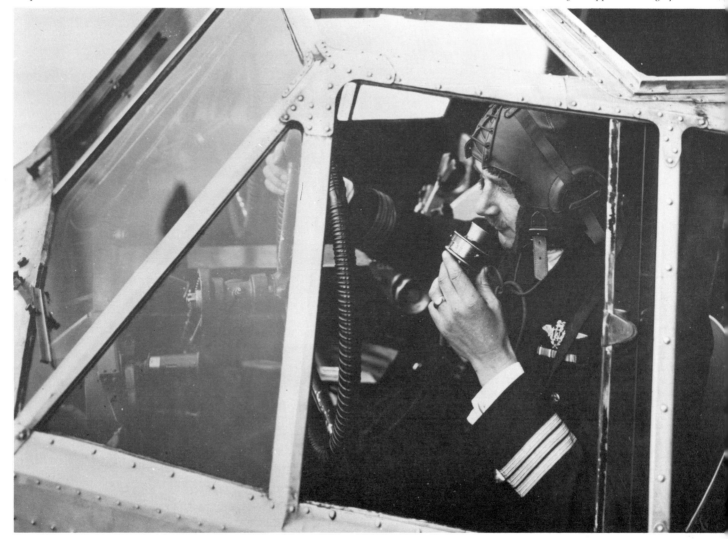

A distinctly unorthodox method of using Gosport tubes for communication was related by a famous Battle of Britain fighter pilot who started his flying career after World War I. When flying with an unpleasant character the trick was to let him know that you had a message for him, quickly relieve oneself down the tube and hold the tube into the slipstream – a sure way of making enemies. Gosport tubes for communication between pilot and observer, passenger or pupil were later replaced by an electric intercom system using a microphone incorporated in the mask or on a strap round the neck and telephones in the helmet.

Communication between two people in an aircraft was one thing but between two aircraft in flight or between an aircraft and the control tower was a different matter. From early this century wireless telegraphy using Morse proved to be a practicable method of communicating between a balloon or aeroplane and the ground, but the first time that speech, as opposed to Morse, was sent from an aircraft in flight to the ground was in 1915. Radio telephony was successfully used on a small scale during World War I, and when the airship R34 crossed the Atlantic in 1919 it was able to remain in radio contact throughout the flight by means of wireless telegraphy and a radio telephone which had a range of fifty miles. A year later, Handley Page Transport, one of the world's first commercial airlines, installed R/T equipment in its Handley Page 0/400 and used it on a flight between Cricklewood and Paris. Initially the adoption of radio telephony was relatively slow, for the equipment was heavy and its use not considered vital. But at the 1925 Hendon Air Display a new and important demonstration took place when nine Gloster Grebes from No 25 Squadron executed co-ordinated formation manoeuvres directed by King George V and others from the ground. This was the first time that radio telephony had been used to control fighter aircraft from the ground. Before its advent the orders of the leader were transmitted to other pilots of the formation by hand signals or special movements of the leader's aircrat.

Radio telephony was widely used during the twenties and thirties by commercial airlines, and by 1932 Imperial Airways aircraft on the Cairo–Cape Town route were able to transmit messages by this means over a range of up to 5,000 miles. But although radio telephony had been used by the RAF since the war it was not widely adopted until the latter part of the 1930s. Military fighter aircraft such as the Hart were equipped with the Morse key, whereas bombers such as the Heyford and Hendon used telephonic communication which was operated by a wireless operator with a hand microphone. A hand microphone was suitable for certain crew members but it was much easier for a pilot if the microphone was incorporated in the mask, so that he could keep his hands free to control the aircraft.

More new equipment

The Mk I mask, which was obsolete by 1921, and the Mk II mask were both basic oxygen masks, but by 1921 a fur-lined helmet was available with a detachable oxygen-breathing mask that could be adapted for use with wireless receivers and wireless telephone receivers and transmitters. The mask was much the same shape as the Mks I and II, covering the nose, cheeks, mouth and chin, but was of black leather edged with fur and instead of being held on by an elastic strap round the back of the head it was attached by lacing to the right of the cap and by a strap and buckle to the left. The Types A, B and C masks worn during the early thirties were of much the same design as before, although without the fur edging, but unlike the Mks I and II a cap could be removed from the conical dome at the front of the mask and a microphone of a diameter of about two and a half inches fitted. The masks were attached to the 1930 flying helmet by leather straps and buckles rather than by an elastic strap.

The Type B mask introduced in 1933 was used until 1939. Made of brown water proof twill lined with linen, it had a chamois-covered cap which could be removed for the fitting of a microphone if required. But in 1936 a new helmet and mask were introduced, for high-altitude flights. They were the Type B helmet and Type D mask which, instead of being attached to each other by straps and buckles, were fitted together with four snap fasteners. The latter were better able to support the weight of microphone cords and oxygen tubing. There was a quick-release strap under the chin and a strap at the back of

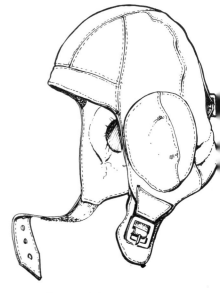

1930 Pattern helmet. 22C/51. Made of chestnut brown chrome leather, this helmet was a forerunner of the B Type and superseded the MKI helmet; it was elasticated at the back to suit individual wearers. Earpads had small shallow sockets to allow the fitting of telephones or Gosport Tubes. The leather covering flaps 22C/57 over the ears were held with press studs.

the helmet which could be tightened to ensure a well fitting helmet and mask. The Type B helmet and Type D mask were worn with the Mk IIIA goggles. The helmet had zipped, leather-covered, padded earpieces shaped like doughnuts and was in use during the early years of World War II. Soft leather face-protectors snapped inside the helmet when the mask was not in use to prevent the metal fasteners from freezing onto the face.

Face masks had been used since the earliest flying days to protect the wearer from the agonies of frostbite, but towards the end of World War I the face mask had been adapted to incorporate oxygen-breathing and communications equipment. Whereas during the wartime years oxygen equipment had not been available to all RAF pilots, this situation was now changed, but because the equipment was of a rather unreliable and primitive nature most flights did not exceed 10,000ft, a height at which reasonable efficiency without oxygen can be maintained. Most flights exceeding this height tended to be of an experimental nature or else they were meteorological flights to check weather conditions.

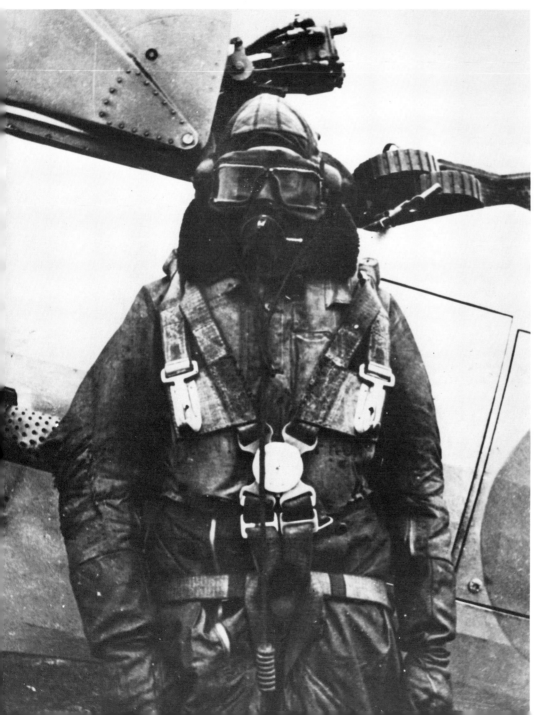

A rear-gunner of a Hawker Demon wearing a 1930 pattern suit, a B Type helmet seemingly inside out, D Type mask, MKIIIA goggles and the early pattern life preserver. The parachute harness is designed to take a chest pack.

The Mk I oxygen mask, as mentioned in the previous chapter, and its successors, the Mk II and Types A, B, C and D masks during the inter-war years, all relied on a continuous-flow system of delivery; but since inhalation extends over rather less than half the breathing cycle at least half the oxygen supplied flowed to waste during exhalation. The method was therefore extremely wasteful because twice as much oxygen was delivered as was needed. There were manually controlled rates of flow which were altered with altitude, but the system was very arbitrary. Furthermore, the masks fitted badly and were uncomfortable. Although much work was being done in this period on improved methods of delivering oxygen, the continuous-flow system was used until 1942.

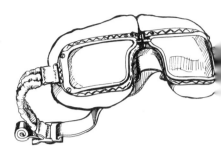

Immediately after World War I both liquid and compressed gaseous oxygen were being used in aircraft. The advantages of the former were that it was safer to use under rifle- and shell-fire, that, unlike gaseous oxygen, it was free of moisture which could freeze and block the tube, and that the containers weighed very much less than high-pressure oxygen cylinders for an equivalent capacity. They were therefore more suitable for use on long-range reconnaissance or bomber flights. Potentially, liquid oxygen was of greatest use overseas, but owing to problems of storage, supply and transport its advantages were minimal. The pipe-stem mouthpiece through which oxygen was inhaled was a tiring contraption to use since it had to be gripped constantly between the teeth, and therefore users tended to develop a stiff jaw. As a result much precious oxygen was wasted. By 1930 the use of liquid oxygen in aircraft had been phased out.

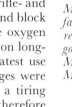

MKIIIA goggles are perhaps the most famous. Introduced in 1933, they were not replaced until the introducton of the MKI goggles in August 1940 and the subsequent MKVII a year later. Like the Goggles Mask MKII, the MKIIIs had single lenses.

The acceptance of the parachute

Another piece of standard equipment to be introduced in the inter-war years was the parachute. Since 1916 Ernest Calthrop, the inventor of the unwieldy Guardian Angel static-line parachute, had been desperately trying to interest the Air Ministry in his design. It was developed on a very limited scale in 1919 for use in Avro training aircraft, but four years later was declared obsolete. The great turning-point came in 1925 when the American-designed Irvin 'free-fall' parachute was adopted as standard equipment for all aircrew, and a Parachute Training Unit was established at Henlow, in Bedfordshire. At last parachutes were no longer the prerogative of a favoured few; the Air Ministry had tardily decided to follow the good examples of Germany and later America in making 'chutes standard issue. It now remained only for the old wicker or leather aircraft seats to be replaced by specially designed metal ones. To prevent a pilot from having to bend virtually double when sitting on a seat-type pack in his aircraft, a special recess was built into the seat to incorporate the pack. The static-line parachute was used during the inter-war years by balloonists who wore a parachute pack attached by a rope to the balloon basket. This meant that when the balloonist jumped, the correct length of line operated the parachute automatically. In this way the parachute opened rapidly, a matter of vital importance to balloonists, who tended to operate at lower altitudes. Manually operated parachutes were used by all other airmen as they offered much greater flexibility. In an emergency an airman could jump from any exit in the aircraft and, if jumping at great altitudes, could free-fall at high speed through the thin, cold atmosphere before operating the 'chute. Static-line parachutes in aircraft necessitated jumping from the exit closest to where the line was attached, and this could prove extremely difficult if the aircraft was in an unusual position. In the 1930s the all-British GQ firm, named after its two directors, James Gregory and Raymond Quilter, introduced a new type of parachute in which the shroud lines were kept in vanes to prevent fouling, and which had a cup-shaped canopy producing minimal oscillation. The parachute was widely used and by 1930 fifty-two servicemen had qualified for the famous 'golden caterpillar' tie-pin, and the number of unpremeditated descents increased steadily.

There were four basic types of parachute pack: the seat, lap, chest and back, all of which clipped on to the webbing harness worn on top of the flying clothing. Pilots and crew members who had no need to move around inside the aircraft used a seat-type pack which was permanently clipped on to the harness and acted as a cushion. By 1936 all aircraft seats were specially designed to take a seat-type pack. Before this date some pilots, for example in Fairey Flycatchers, had to use back-type packs as the seat could not be lowered far enough to accommodate a seat pack. To add to the Flycatcher pilot's difficulties, the cockpit opening was so small that it was impossible to get in or out when wearing a parachute. The problem of getting in could be solved by putting the pack in first but getting out was a very different matter. In an emergency there was no way that a pilot could attach the pack to his harness and hope to leave the aircraft. He would simply have got stuck. Yet the only alternative, that of getting the pack and yourself out separately and then hoping to attach the pack to the harness while plumetting earthwards must have been a hair-raising prospect. The cockpit of the Handley Page Heyford was so cramped that the pilot was unable to wear a parachute at all and had to stow it elsewhere. They used two-point detachable chest-type packs which could be easily clipped on to the harness. But in a moment of crisis the Heyford pilot had actually to leave the controls and the cockpit to retrieve his parachute.

What the well-dressed test pilot wore in 1929. Herb Fahy, a Lockheed test pilot.

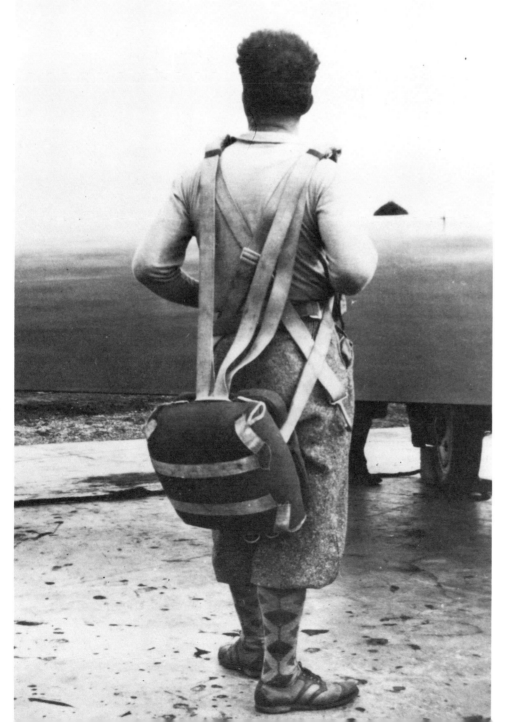

Harnesses

At the beginning of the inter-war period observers and gunners used back-packs which were extremely uncomfortable when the wearer was standing up in the slipstream. Lap-type packs were then introduced and later the two-point detachable chest-type, which was stowed near the airman and quickly clipped on when required, thus avoiding the extra weight, bulk and discomfort. The parachute harness was also used to attach a fighting harness known as a 'monkey chain', from the observer or gunner to the aircraft. This ensured his safety when having to stand up and perform his job while the aircraft was flying. Back-packs were used for training purposes, along with a small reserve pack on the chest. They were also used by airship crews, who stowed the harness and pack together in an accessible place, using a strip of aluminium to keep the harness open. Prominently placed sheath knives could be used to cut through the airship's envelope in an emergency.

In the early 1930s a single-point, quick-release harness was introduced for all airmen engaged in marine operations so that they could instantaneously release themselves from the parachute after descending into water. Before this date parachutes were not favoured by the Admiralty because, if the parachute did not release easily, the airman could be dragged down by the canopy and drowned. In 1932 a standard, inflatable life-saving waistcoat of stole pattern, the forerunner of the Mae West, was introduced, replacing the various patterns of life-saving jacket, waistcoat and belt then in use; but even this was unable to keep afloat someone who was attached to a large, heavy, sinking mass of parachute. These life-jackets were of a grey/green colour and contained kapok pads which kept the wearer afloat while he inflated the stole. CO_2 canisters were not introduced until the early years of the war.

A major invention which appeared four years later in 1936 was the combined flying suit, parachute harness and life-saving waistcoat manufactured by the Irvin Company for pilots and crews of flying boats. It consisted of an outer flying suit into which was fitted a lining carrying a parachute harness as well as a safety harness for connection to the observer's anchorage. The sleeveless lining made of khaki cloth was attached to the outer suit by buttons and had legs that terminated below the knees. A gas-inflated, life-saving stole was fitted inside the suit, but over the lining, and was constructed of several layers of rubberised silk fabric. The parachute pack was of a two-point detachable type.

Another life-saving device which, although not flying clothing as such did impose restrictions on the pilot's body, was the safety harness. The Sutton harness had been introduced towards the end of World War I. Consisting of four lengths of webbing, two of which passed over the pilot's shoulders and two over his thighs, it held the pilot firmly in his seat during inverted flight as well as on impact with the ground, could be quickly released in an emergency and was adjustable to any size. It was a great advance on its predecessor, the lap-type belt, which was extremely dangerous in inverted flight, often snapped on impact and, even if it held firm, it did not prevent the upper part of the pilot's body from being flung forward. But the Sutton harness was mistakenly regarded primarily as a safety device in dog-fights and not considered a necessity for peacetime flying.

For several years after the war many aircraft were fitted with the lap-belt, a cause of a large proportion of injuries. The Siskin was a difficult aircraft to land, often pitching forward on to its nose and throwing the pilot against the instrument panel. It was claimed that many former Siskin pilots had acquired a distinctive Roman nose known as the Siskin nose, as a result of such an accident. In 1921 forty-three Sutton Harnesses were issued for use in Snipe aircraft and two years later 125 of them for single-seater fighter aircraft. It was not, however, until about 1928 that Sutton harnesses became a standard safety measure. The development of aerobatics and the increased performance of fighter aircraft necessitated a more serious policy towards the use of harnesses. The only possible drawback of the Sutton quick-release harness was when an aircraft turned upside-down on landing. If the pilot of a biplane in this situation rather absent-mindedly pulled the quick-release catch he would fall several feet to the ground. On numerous occasions pilots owed their lives to the harness but were often pulled away from the aircraft concussed or unconscious because they had undone the harness without due thought.

Cabins and cockpits

The discomforts experienced when flying in an open-cockpit aircraft were greatly relieved by the introduction of the enclosed cockpit, an inter-war design advance that had a noticeable effect on the type of clothing worn in flight. Commercial aviation, ever conscious of the passengers' comforts, was the first to introduce the enclosed cabin as a feasible proposition. Immediately after the war converted military aircraft had been used for the transportation of civilians. The journeys were usually lengthy and hazardous. A passenger was provided with layers of protective clothing, given a hot-water bottle and squashed into the observer's seat. The *Aeroplane* records the aerial journey in 1919 from Paris to London of an American and an Irish priest. Aided by a strong tail-wind and a bottle of cognac they arrived home in a record one and three-quarter hours, only to discover that the American's bowler hat had been flattened in the vicious slipstream, its brim having firmly wedged itself round his chin.

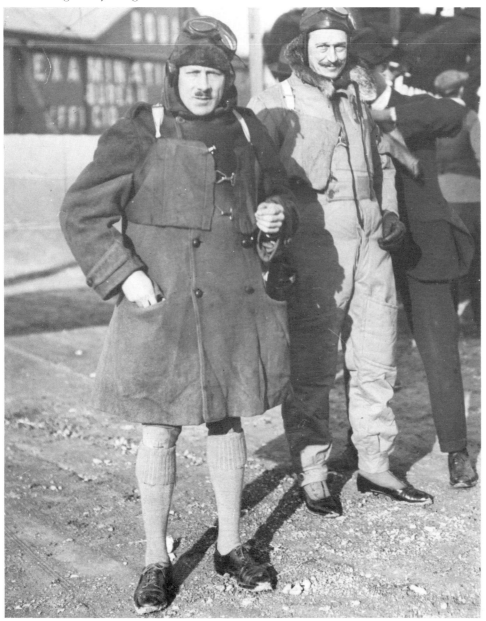

Pilots about to embark on a cross-Channel commercial flight from Hounslow Heath, c. 1920.
Both are wearing inflatable life-jackets.

Within a few years, aircraft such as the de Havilland DH34 provided an enclosed cabin for the passengers, although the pilot was still exposed to the icy slipstream in order, it was argued, to keep him awake. Passengers no longer had to be clad in a leather coat, helmet and goggles, although travelling rugs and foot muffs helped keep out draughts, and a warm coat was always advisable. Many unfortunate passengers suffered severe air-sickness resulting from a combination of nerves, incessant noise, vibration and turbulence. Pots were suitably positioned under the seats and cotton wool provided to deaden the roar of the engines. Until sound-proofing was introduced the noise was such that one had difficulty in conversing with one's next-door neighbour. Furthermore, because at this date cabins were unpressurised, any noticeable change of altitude caused one's ears to 'pop', often with great discomfort. Over the years the interior design of passenger aircraft improved. Seating arrangements progressed from the upright wicker seat to the soft upholstered seat, and adequate heating and ventilation were soon provided. Even today people look back longingly to the steadfast aeroplanes and romantic flying boats of Imperial Airways and to the days of the luxurious Zeppelin airships which floated majestically across the Atlantic.

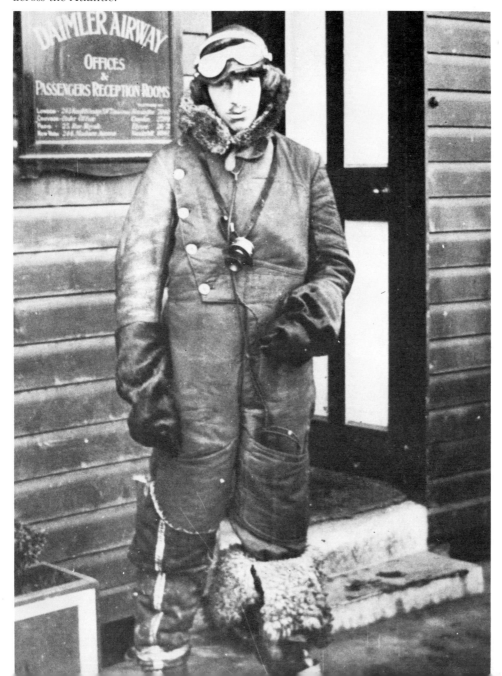

An early style airline pilot wearing a Sidcot suit, goggle mask Mk I and cut down 'fug' boots.

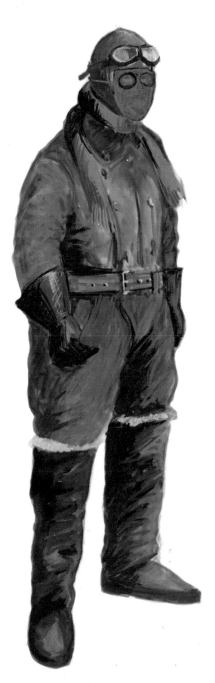

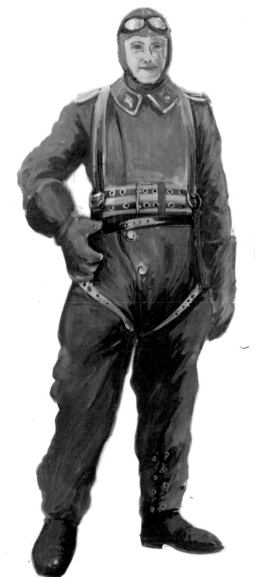

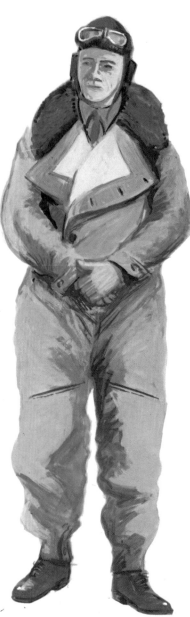

A pilot of the Imperial Air Service (German) in 1916. He wears a one piece flying suit, type unknown as outfitting was left largely to the individual. However the goggles and overboots appear so often they may well have been issue items.
The face mask was a common do it yourself piece of equipment often made from pigskin as is this flying helmet.

An Imperial Air Service pilot in 1918 wearing a Heinecke parachute harness, grey greatcoat tucked into Fleigerhosen which were issued. The harness was strengthened with leather and later harnesses were reinforced as the result of early failures. The pilot wears the earlier harness with narrow leg straps.

A Royal Flying Corps pilot wearing a Sidcot Suit, Mk.I flying helmet and a Triplex Mk.I goggle mask. This outfit with gauntlets was fairly standard after the Sidcot suit became available in March 1918.

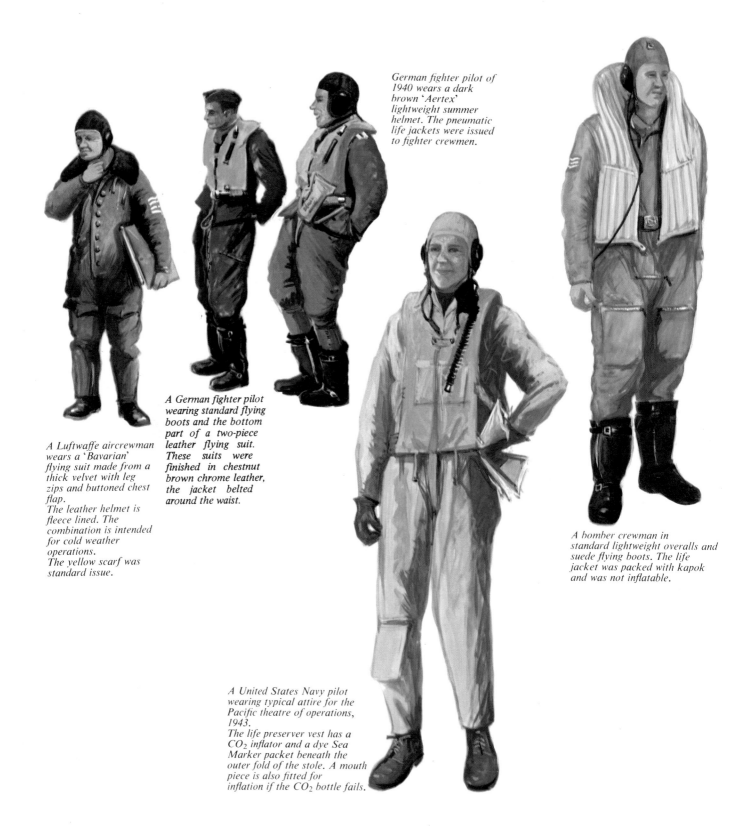

German fighter pilot of 1940 wears a dark brown 'Aertex' lightweight summer helmet. The pneumatic life jackets were issued to fighter crewmen.

A Luftwaffe aircrewman wears a 'Bavarian' flying suit made from a thick velvet with leg zips and buttoned chest flap.
The leather helmet is fleece lined. The combination is intended for cold weather operations.
The yellow scarf was standard issue.

A German fighter pilot wearing standard flying boots and the bottom part of a two-piece leather flying suit. These suits were finished in chestnut brown chrome leather, the jacket belted around the waist.

A bomber crewman in standard lightweight overalls and suede flying boots. The life jacket was packed with kapok and was not inflatable.

A United States Navy pilot wearing typical attire for the Pacific theatre of operations, 1943.
The life preserver vest has a CO_2 inflator and a dye Sea Marker packet beneath the outer fold of the stole. A mouth piece is also fitted for inflation if the CO_2 bottle fails.

Passengers could tolerate being airsick and shivery, bumping along at a few thousand feet above the earth, but when the DC3s started to fly above 10,000ft, passing *over* high terrain rather than *round* it, and oxygen masks were introduced, they felt that this was the limit; not only was it unnerving but also uncomfortable. While the aircraft was above 10,000ft passengers were not allowed to smoke, had difficulty in eating and drinking, and a visit to the lavatory was impossible without an extended oxygen lead. As this was never introduced they had to sit tight. It was not until aircraft were pressurised that this problem was solved.

The Handley Page HP42 introduced in 1931 was one of the first aircraft to give the pilot as well as his passengers a modicum of comfort by enclosing the cockpit. No longer did he have to suffer from watering eyes as the wind crept round his goggles, from the chilling blast of the slipstream, or from cold, sodden clothing after passing through a rain storm. He discarded his goggles and leather protective clothing for a prestigious blue serge uniform sporting gold braid, and a peaked cap, and as a result was now regarded by his passengers with much greater respect if not actually held in awe. The enclosed cockpit was a great innovation that alleviated if not eliminated many miseries the pilot had formerly to endure.

Inside a de Havilland Dragon.

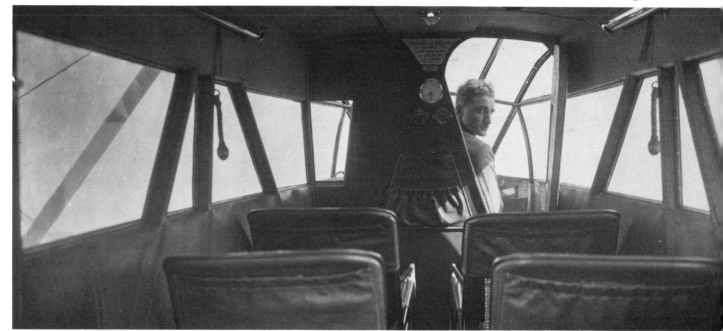

It took rather longer for these bonuses to reach the military pilot. He had to grin and bear it for several years more. The mid-upper gunner of the Handley Page Heyford was semi-protected by a propped flap, as were certain crew members of the Fairey Hendon, the first monoplane bomber; the speed of the Hawker Hart Bomber, in excess of the current fighters, led to the development of a fighter version, the Hawker Demon, which had a lobster-back turret designed to protect the gunner. The slipstream was extremely fierce and made the changing of ammunition drums on the machine gun almost impossible without some protection. The Boulton Paul Overstrand, one of the most advanced aircraft of its kind, boasted a power-operated, enclosed gun-turret in the nose, and enclosed cockpit for the pilot, heating for the crew and a large protective windscreen for the mid-upper gunner, but this was not in full production until 1935 and only one squadron was thus equipped. The Westland Wallace II of the same date had an enclosed cockpit for pilot and observer. The first RAF aircraft that provided complete protection for all the crew was the well-loved Avro Anson which was in operational service from 1936.

The Hawker Hurricane was the first monoplane fighter in RAF service. It was designed with an enclosed cockpit and although it flew twice as fast as many contemporary aircraft types the pilot required less clothing because of the canopy which protected him against the effects of slipstream and cold.

Pioneering

Generally speaking, the design of everyday flying clothing evolved gradually. Additional press-studs, pockets, seams and stitches appeared, different materials were introduced, but revolutionary innovations were few and far between. White overalls became the new trademark of the inter-war period for civilian and serviceman alike, the Sidcot-pattern suit was available to all airmen, and airline pilots now wore smart uniforms; parachutes, radio telephony and oxygen equipment were generally used, but standard inter-war clothing was not radically different from that worn towards the end of World War I.

It was in the realms of record-breaking, of flying higher, faster and further than before, that new clothing problems arose and where innovations were necessary. The innumerable, pioneering long-distance flights which paved the way for the civil air routes of today and contributed greatly to the techniques of aerial navigation imposed an enormous physical and psychological strain on the pilot and his crew. In 1919, the year that Alcock and Brown flew the Atlantic, Ross and Keith Smith, J. M. Bennett and W. H. Shiers set off in a Vickers Vimy from Hounslow to Australia. They crossed the Channel in dense cumulo-nimbus and a blinding snowstorm, and on ascending to 9,000 ft in the hopes of rising above the bad weather the aircraft's wings and the crew's goggles iced up. After six hours in such conditions the crew were numb with cold and even their sandwiches had frozen solid. When crossing the Appennines the Vimy encountered turbulence which tossed the aircraft up and down like a small boat in a storm. They were later caught in a torrential rain storm, were soaked to the skin and could see nothing with their goggles on, yet were blinded by the rain if they took them off. Poor Ross Smith wrote, 'This sort of flying is a rotten game. The cold is hell and I am silly for having ever embarked on the flight.' They covered the 11,000 miles in almost twenty-one days.

Sir Sefton Brancker and his pilot Alan Cobham, the famous pioneer of airline routes, about to embark on a route survey from London to India, November 1924.

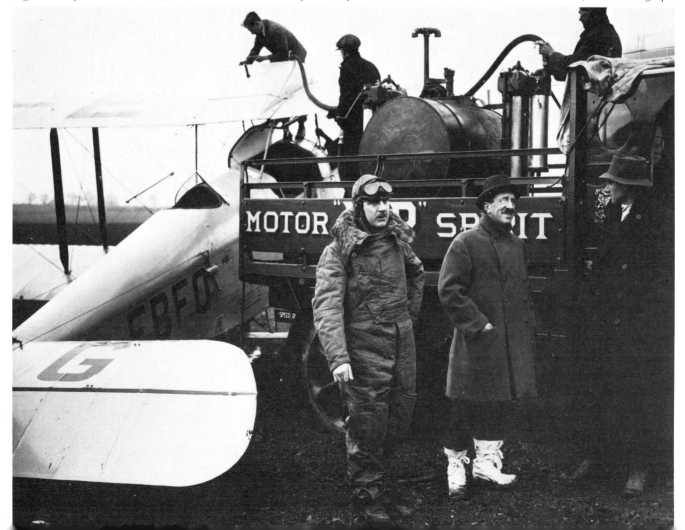

In the twenties Alan Cobham made his famous pioneering flights to Cairo, India, Australia and South Africa. In 1926 Richard Byrd made the first flight over the North Pole, protected by an Eskimo parka made of reindeer skin which was warm in temperatures as low as −60°C and which had a hood lined with wolverine – a fur which repels ice and snow. Two enemies in Polar regions are moisture, which causes frostbite, and wind which exacerbates the bitter cold. Body temperature decreases much more rapidly in windy conditions even when the temperature is slightly above zero than it does with no wind when the temperature is well below zero. Many layers of underclothing were necessary to trap the warm air. Two years after Byrd's flight Umberto Nobile and his crew flew the ill-fated airship *Italia* to the North Pole. Their clothing consisted of lambswool suits with the fur on the inside and the wind and water-proofed skin on the outside, reindeer-skin parkas, sealskin trousers and oversize sealskin boots lined with carex grass for insulation. In flight they wore lambswool slippers inside reindeer-skin shoes instead of the unwieldy sealskin boots. The total outfit weighed approximately twelve pounds, somewhat restricting ease and rapidity of movement.

In 1930 Amy Johnson flew solo to Australia in nineteen days, and two years later Amelia Earhart made the first solo crossing of the Atlantic by a woman. In 1933 two RAF officers, Gayford and Nicoletts, flew over 5,000 miles to South-West Africa in a Fairey long-range monoplane establishing a world long-distance record. Weight restrictions on such flights were stringent yet it was insisted that they take their mess kits so that they could appear decently attired when entertained on arrival. One of the main problems encountered in long-distance flying is that of overcoming fatigue. Charles Lindbergh had not slept for sixty-three hours by the time he had completed his 33 hour Atlantic solo flight in 1927. In 1933 Wiley post embarked on the first solo flight around the world. In practising to overcome the problem of fatigue he would never sleep the same hours on any two nights of the week.

Amy Johnson prior to her flight to Capetown, 1932.

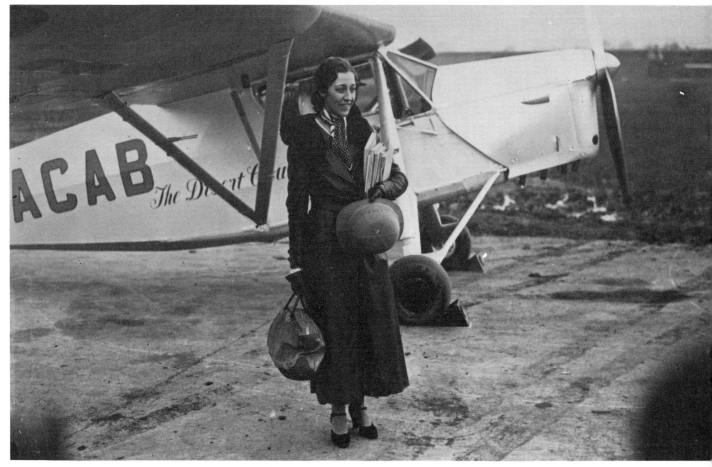

High altitude, low temperature

Special equipment had to be developed for the first flight over Mount Everest, in 1933. Flying in two Westland open-cockpit aircraft the main danger for the crew was that their goggles would ice over and that their vital oxygen equipment would also freeze. Special goggles were designed by Messrs James Stephens unobtrusively incorporating thin electric filaments between two layers of perspex. Without this aid the venture would have been impossible, for to fly without goggles at that altitude would have frozen the crews' eyeballs, but visibility with goggles covered with thick layers of ice would have been nil. The oxygen supply could have been similarly affected for the smallest amount of moisture present in the supply would freeze and block the tiny orifice in the regulating valve. The oxygen had therefore to be electrically heated on its way to the crews' masks. Failure of this system would have resulted in certain anoxia and death. The aviators wore inner suits designed by Siebe-Gorman and Company. These were made of quilted kapok incorporating a mass of heating wires. The outer suit was of a thick wind-proof material which zipped up the front. The sheepskin flying boots and gloves were also heated in a similar fashion, while silk inner gloves facilitated the rapid and precise handling of switches and instruments.

The special goggles used for the flight over Everest.

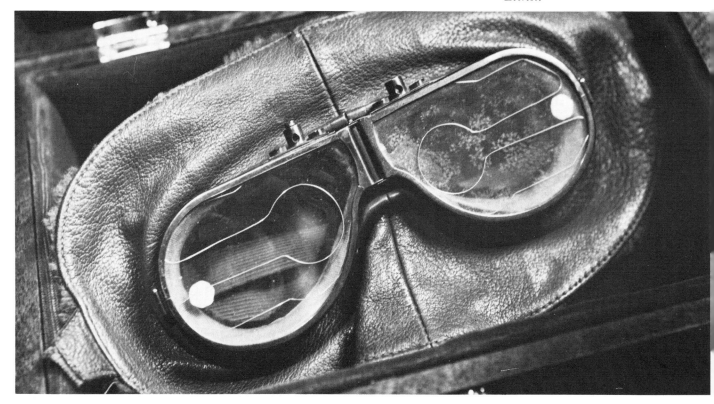

Similar adventures occurred four years later, in 1937, when three Russians, Baidukov, Chkalov and Beliakov flew over 5,500 miles from Moscow to Seattle via the North Pole in an ANT25. Ill-equipped with oxygen and clothing, they flew for more than sixty-two hours. Clad in silk underwear, woollen sweaters, leather breeches lined with eiderdown, and reindeer boots they sometimes had to withstand temperatures of −30°C. With no electrically heated clothing, and with a cabin heater that had little effect at any altitude the conditions were appalling. Their oxygen supply soon began to run out when, to avoid the wings icing up, they flew for long periods at great altitudes, above the weather. When crossing the Rocky Mountains at 20,000 ft, Chkalov's nose started to bleed into his oxygen mask, and after desperate rationing of oxygen the supply ran out. Miraculously they lived to tell the tale.

Speed and strain

As with long-distance flights, so with speed-record-breaking attempts very real strains were put on the human body. Any constant speed in straight and level flight does not affect the pilot, but rapid acceleration or deceleration in any direction can cause the pilot to black out; for during tight turns or rapid manoeuvres blood drains from the brain into the abdomen and legs. This problem of 'G' did not occur on any widespread scale until World War II, for until that date few aircraft, other than special racing aircraft, were designed to withstand such forces.

Flying Officer Waghorn being helped ashore after a trial flight for the Schneider Trophy, 1929.

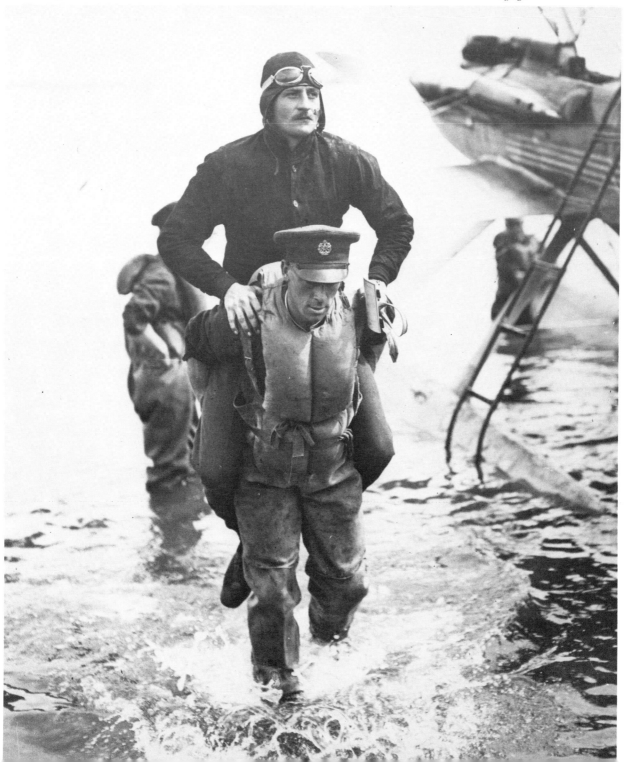

Within a few years aircraft performances had improved greatly. The Supermarine S4 established a speed record of 227 mph in the 1925 Schneider Trophy. Britain won the trophy outright in 1931 with the S6B at a speed of 340 mph, and later that year it attained a world speed record of 407 mph. Special goggles were designed for the British contestants for the 1927 Schneider Trophy because it was found that the slipstream entered the ventilation holes of the standard-issue goggles, making their eyes water so much they could barely see. The competitors in the Schneider Trophy seaplane speed race had to withstand a certain amount of 'G' if they took the corners on the triangular course too sharply. Early suggestions for the solution of this problem were, for example, that the pilot shout during the pull-out, that he crouch (which would prove tricky if he was strapped in), that oxygen be used as a stimulant, or that an abdominal belt inflated from an airstream intake be used to prevent blood from being forced down the body. The Americans insisted that terminal velocity dives were made with all fighter aircraft they intended to purchase. To avoid black-outs pilots even tried tying a silk scarf tightly round their necks for the few moments necessary for this manoeuvre, the idea being to staunch the flow of blood away from the brain when the positive 'G' forces of a pull-out were applied. As early as 1934 the Germans were using a centrifuge to test the effects of acceleration on the human body, but no real solution to these problems was found until World War II.

Pressurisation

But from the flying clothing point of view the high-altitude experiments of the inter-war years were most significant. Balloons paved the way in the field of high-altitude flight. In the late 1920s ascents were made to as much as 40,000 ft in open gondolas. Ascents much above this height proved fatal, and it was a Swiss Professor, Auguste Piccard, who realised that the answer lay in developing a gondola that was not only fully enclosed but also pressurised so that the temperature, pressure and oxygen content of the air were regulated. In 1935 a pressurised gondola took two Americans to an amazing record height of 72,395 ft. The idea of taking life-sustaining atmosphere to conquer the hostile regions of the stratosphere was later developed with pressurised heavier-than-air craft in the early years of the war. Until this date relatively few aircraft other than the odd record-breaking, high-altitude flights penetrated the stratosphere (above approximately 36,000 ft). Meteorological flights, however, would often be carried out up to heights of 22,000 ft, where warm clothing would be essential and oxygen vital. But the development in the 1930s of superchargers greatly increased aircraft ceilings, for by compressing the air entering the carburettor they maintained sea-level air density in the engine's induction system, allowing it to give full power, even in rarefied air. In 1932 Captain Cyril F. Uwins of the RAF in an open-cockpit aircraft reached 43,976 ft, a height at which, in the standard atmosphere, the temperature would have been at least $-56°C$. The record that stood during the war years was the one established by the Italian Colonel Mario Pezzi who, in 1938, reached a height of 56,046 ft in a turbo-charged Caproni 151.

Although an oxygen supply is necessary above 14,000 ft, above 40,000 ft man also needs artificial pressure to force this oxygen into his lungs and bloodstream, since at that height the air pressure is less than one-fifth of that at sea-level. The solution is therefore either to pressurise the whole cockpit or gondola or else to breathe oxygen under pressure. Simply to force pressurised oxygen into the pilot's lungs through an oxygen mask would at high altitude cause him to balloon outwards. The internal pressure of oxygen must be equalised by a similar external force. The solution of the inter-war years was the development of an all-enveloping pressurised suit and mask so that atmospheric conditions similar to those at sea-level could be artificially maintained. The concept of a pressure suit originated with an English respiratory physiologist J. S. Haldane who, in 1907, developed a method of gradual decompression making it possible for deep-sea divers to ascend to the surface safely. In 1934 the American pilot Wiley Post became the first man to fly in an aeroplane wearing a pressure suit. The suit was made of an inner 'rubber bag' that contained the gas and an outer layer that maintained the suit's shape. No movable joints were incorporated, and the whole was extremely hot, uncomfortable and unwieldy.

France, Germany, Russia and Italy also tried to develop a fully pressurised suit. Germany had commissioned manufacturers of diving equipment, Drägerwerke of Lübeck, to make a full pressure suit, but it proved most unwieldy. A pressure suit was developed in Germany for high-altitude bale-out but when it was inflated the pilot was unable to sit down! Problems of ballooning, great heat, lack of mobility and joint leakage encouraged these countries to turn more to the development of pressurised cabins as a viable alternative. In 1936 Squadron Leader F. Swain of the Royal Air Force broke the altitude record for heavier-than-air craft when he reached 49,967 ft in the Bristol 138A. His pressure suit, manufactured by Siebe-Gorman, the firm that normally made diving suits, was made of rubberised fabric in two pieces. The trousers were fitted at the waist by a rubber ring to which the upper portion of the suit was attached by means of a flexible steel band. The helmet, made of the same rubberised fabric, incorporated a curved visor of two layers of 'celestoid' between which an air space was dehumidified (to prevent fogging) by means of a drying tube. Pressurised oxygen was circulated round the suit, and through a soda-lime canister so that water vapour and carbon dioxide could be absorbed; fresh oxygen was added as required.

Fl. Lt. Adam.

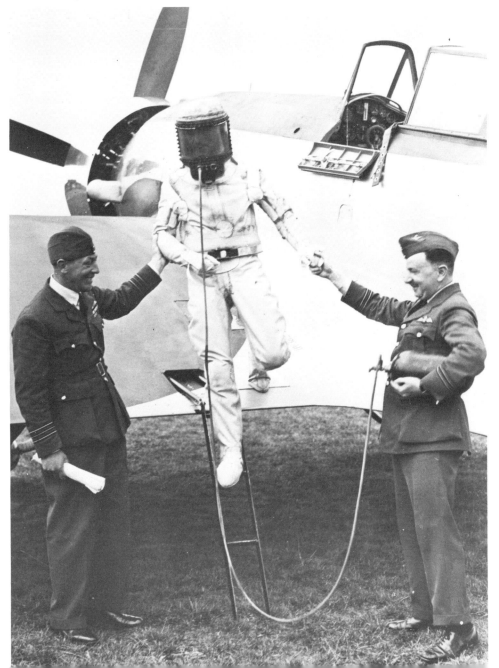

To date the design of full-pressure suits had almost completely sacrificed mobility in order to deliver enough oxygen under pressure to maintain life at very high altitudes. Swain needed several men to help him out to the aircraft and hoist him aboard. In 1937 Flight Lieutenant Adam reached 53,937 ft in the Bristol 138 monoplane wearing a pressure suit very similar to Squadron Leader Swain's, but again it was an extremely lengthy job getting dressed. No provision had been made for sweat evaporation, the view through the visor was limited and, worse still, the windows used to mist up. When the suit was blown up the arms and legs were immobilised, and the headpiece was not detachable. Refinements were obviously vital if the pressure suit was to be more widely adopted.

A pilot's mobility was greatly increased by pressurising the aircraft rather than him. The pressurised cockpit for military aircraft was introduced at a later date; apart from aircraft like the Ju86R, the B29, the Mosquito XVI, the Wellington V and VI and the Spitfire Mk VI, military aircraft were not pressurised until the post-war jet era. But by the late 1930s much work was being done on pressurised cabins for commercial aircraft. It was advantageous for long-distance traffic to fly at high altitudes, partly to be able to fly over the weather, and partly so as to fly at greater speed in the less dense atmosphere. At these altitudes pressurisation was necessary for passenger comfort and eliminated the need for the passengers to wear oxygen masks. The Boeing 307 Stratoliner was the first pressurised high-altitude, long-range transport aircraft, used by Pan American Airways. Four were introduced in 1938.

Great strides had undoubtedly been made in the field of commercial aviation. Instead of being bundled into the back seat of a wartime aircraft, passengers could now travel *en masse* in comfort to many corners of the world. The military pilot also was now enclosed, although in less luxurious surroundings, and men enveloped in earth's life-sustaining atmosphere had ascended in balloons and aeroplanes to penetrate the stratosphere. Solutions had been found for many physiological problems encountered in flight, but with the outbreak of World War II and the resultant technological outburst in the field of aviation many new hurdles were to present themselves. The physiologists discovered there was much to do in very little time.

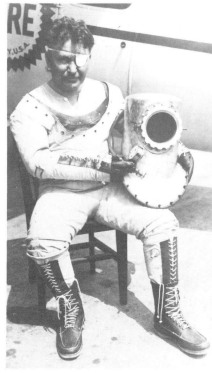

Wiley Post in his third pressure suit.

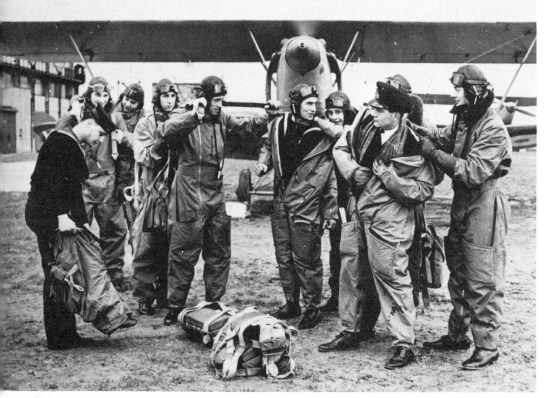

Fleet Air Arm crews in training. The equipment is RAF and basically comprises; 1930 pattern flying suits. Type 'B' helmets adapted for Gosport Tubes, MKIIIA goggles.

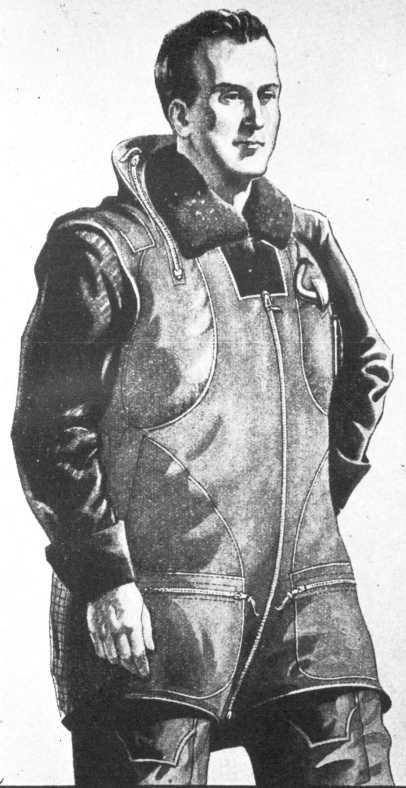

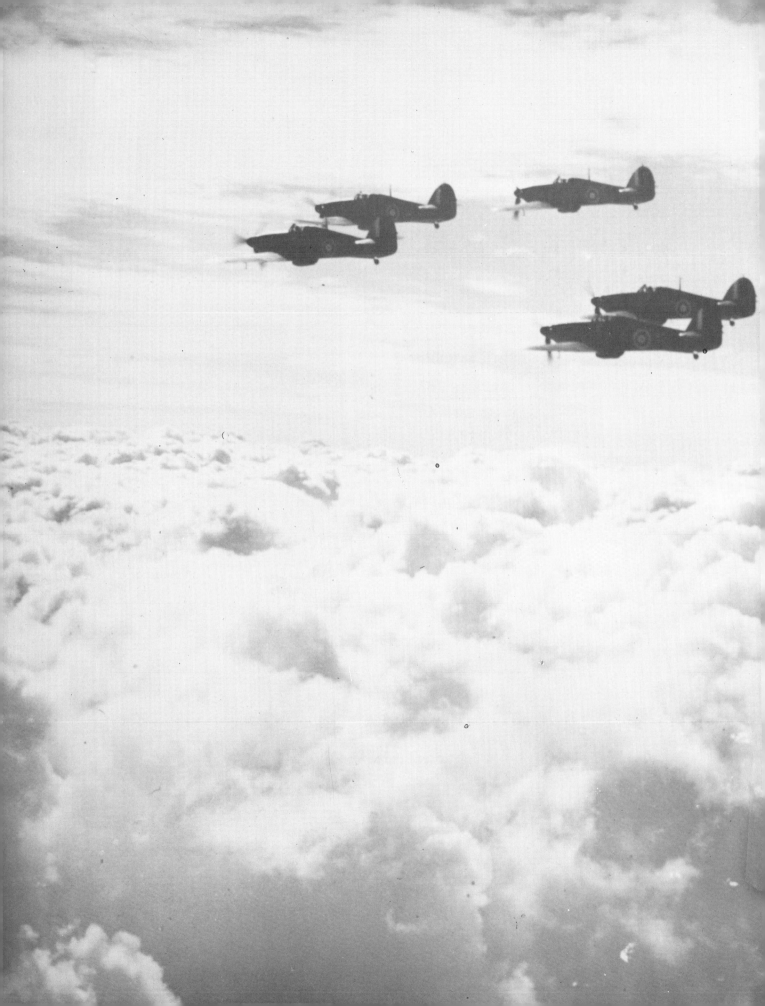

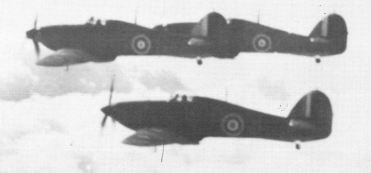

CHAPTER 4
WORLD WAR II—FIGHTER PILOTS

World War II began in September 1939. Within a month the *Luftwaffe* had destroyed the Polish Air Force and marked the way to Warsaw for the German army. Because of defence pacts, Britain found itself at war with Germany. Preparations had been made to increase the size and effectiveness of the Royal Air Force, but these, in retrospect, were left very late. Consequently, when war was declared, the RAF was critically short of front-line aircraft and equipment. Fortunately Britain had eight months' grace, the so-called 'phoney war', when contacts with the enemy were few and she was able to build up the strength of her air force.

In the autumn of 1939 the RAF sent to France an Advanced Air Striking Force (AASF) of Fairey Battles, Blenheims and Hurricanes. The winter weather in Northern France was severe; the warm homeliness of an RAF mess 'somewhere in England' was no longer available. Poorly equipped, with meagre accommodation, the French airfields were unable to offer the British squadrons much in the way of comfort. Huts, tents and houses in the surrounding areas were the refuges for these men.

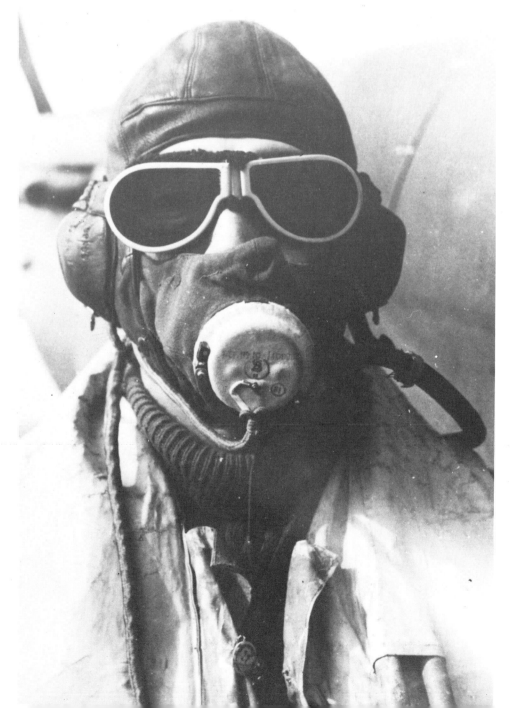

A fighter pilot poses for the camera wearing a 'B' type helmet, 'D' type oxygen mask, MKIII goggle mask and a jacket, life-saving, which has been overpainted yellow.

To combat the cold, aircrew were often to be found wearing their pyjamas and long 'coms' as a foundation for their flying kit proper. The standard-issue kit consisted of a grey/green rubberised 1930-pattern flying suit with a detachable brown fur collar and optional quilted inner lining, or the recently introduced Irvin thermally insulated sheepskin jacket and trousers. Irvin jackets were available with a high, warm collar or alternatively with a form of hood which, when turned inside out, was a bright yellow to aid identification. These two basic outfits were worn immediately over the blue/grey service-dress uniform. The standard-issue flying helmet was the Type B which was designed to accept by means of press-studs the Type D and later the Type F oxygen mask, with or without a microphone fitted. Mk IIIA goggles with the distinctive, oblong-shaped flat lenses were widely used. A little more unusual were the Mk IV and IVA goggles which had a large metal face-plate with split laminated lenses attached to two rubber loops. These loops held fast around the 'doughnut' earpads of the Type B helmet and were kept in place by press-studs attached to the helmets especially for this purpose. The standard flying boot of this period was the 1936-pattern black leather sheepskin-lined boot. The 1932-pattern life-saving waistcoat was worn.

In April 1940 Hitler occupied Norway and Denmark and on 10 May the 'phoney war' in the West came to a sudden halt. Formations of Heinkels, Dorniers and Stukas filled the skies, intent on destroying all military targets in their path. The Germans advanced through the Low Countries and into France, capturing bridges, airfields and important centres of communications. Pilots were forced to flee from airfield to airfield, living in tents or under hedges and fending for themselves. During these weeks many tactical lessons were learned and many heroic actions fought. Six extra squadrons had been sent in May to assist the Advanced Air Striking Force and the Air Component of the Field Force. These squadrons took a considerable toll of enemy aircraft, but with the ground literally being cut beneath them it was only a matter of time before the soil of France would be abandoned. The horrors of murdered refugees lying by the roadsides, the confusion of hastily erected tented accommodation, the burning aircraft and scattered supplies would all be left behind. The evacuation at Dunkirk was the end of the beginning. Hitler's next step would not prove so profitable. This was his attempt to gain air superiority over the Channel in preparation for an invasion of the British Isles. The conflict that ensued was to become known as the Battle of Britain.

Contact with the enemy

Because of its geographical location, south-east England became the target for the full weight of the *Luftwaffe* attack. This attack was intended primarily to reduce airfields, factories and communications to rubble. German fighters were to act in large numbers as escorts for the bomber formations, who would deliver the attacks. However, the German fighters' area of operations was restricted by their fuel-carrying capacity, and the bombers were not well armed; disadvantages which allowed the resources of 11 Group Fighter Command to be used effectively in our defence.

The summer of 1940 was exceptionally hot, and every day massive formations of German bombers and fighters droned across the Channel to do their worst. Flights and Squadrons of RAF fighters patrolled our coastal areas, until vectored by ground radar controllers towards the enemy. Against incredible odds attacks were made to disperse the bomber formations. The Battle of Britain, which began on 8 August, consumed pilots and machines at a prodigious rate. The RAF by the latter part of September 1940 was quite well supplied with aircraft, but was desperately short of experienced fighter pilots. Many were 'rested' in quieter zones of the British Isles after a spell of intense fighting, whilst fresh squadrons were moved into the active zone. Pilots were drawn from re-trained contingents of Poles, Czechoslovaks, Belgians and men from Commonwealth countries, as well as from Army co-operation squadrons.

The average Battle of Britain fighter pilot wore his blue/grey service-dress uniform, a life-saving waistcoat painted yellow which was inflated by the wearer, a Type 'B' leather helmet with padded telephones in the earpieces, Mk IIIA or Mk IV goggles, a Type D green canvas face mask fastened to the helmet by press-studs and fitted with a microphone and oxygen tube. Oxygen was supplied on a constant-flow basis. Flying boots of

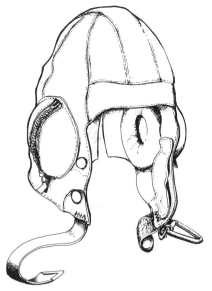

RAF Type B helmet. Introduced in the mid 1930's, it was replaced with the Type C in late 1941. This helmet was designed to take the Type D mask which was tailored to suit the wearer's face. The design of the helmet differed from the 1930 Pattern in as much as zipped earpads were fitted (Ref 22C/66) and the back of the helmet was split. A Bennett quick-release fastener, when pulled tight, closed the gap and also allowed the helmet to be taken off quickly in an emergency. Electrical wiring was external.

the 1936 pattern or the new 1940 pattern were worn; the latter were fleece lined and had black leather shoe bottoms with canvas-covered calves. The 1930- and 1940-pattern flying suits were both available to fighter pilots during the Battle of Britain but it was such a hot summer that these suits were uncomfortable to wear while waiting to scramble. The 1940-pattern flying suit was a very popular introduction for, although almost identical to its predecessor, the 1930-pattern suit, it was made of gabardine rather than a sweaty rubberised fabric. As from the autumn of 1940 it was widely used during the war, and in 1941 a wired, electrically heated version was introduced, also made of a grey/green fabric.

If a pilot was on a chilly dawn patrol he would very often put his flying kit on over his pyjamas with a white polo-necked sweater (Frock White) over his shirt and an Irvin jacket on top of that. The Frock, Aircrew, was described in the RAF magazine *Tee Emm* as 'a cosy woollen confection which turns out to be a sweater built on W. G. Grace lines, in which a small air-gunner can remain decent even when debagged.' It was important to avoid puddles or grass with dew when walking out to the aircraft as the 1940-pattern boots were not water-proof. To fly at altitude wearing wet boots which would probably freeze solid was a certain recipe for severe frostbite. During the Battle of Britain, fighter pilots were very much in the public eye. Many literally dropped in on the end of a parachute. They became national heroes, and much was made of the fact that they were allowed to have the top button of their tunic undone while on duty. But a more significant trait was the use of the Old School cravat or of a silk or woollen scarf tied round the neck and tucked inside the shirt. A fighter pilot once airborne had to be continuously looking around him for enemy aircraft. The scarf prevented his neck from being rubbed raw by a stiff collar. Some pilots, however, did not wear scarves as these could get tangled in the aircraft's controls, and a pilot could be strangled by a loose scarf if caught in a fierce slipstream.

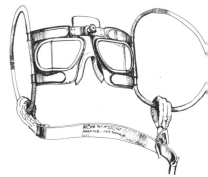

Goggles MKIV. Probably the most complicated of goggles. They required metal plat to aid their attachment to Type B helme. First introduced in August 1940, they wei subsequently replaced by MKVII's. The were the first goggles to feature the sp lenses. Some were available with a separc polarised screen which could be swung dov to shield the eyes from the sun. They had t same attachment to the goggles as t MKVII.

Pilots of 85 Squadron in the summer 1940, including Flt. Lt. Peter Townsen wearing pre-war overalls. They are c wearing the 1932 Pattern life jacket, sen inflated, and some wear 1936 Pattern boo

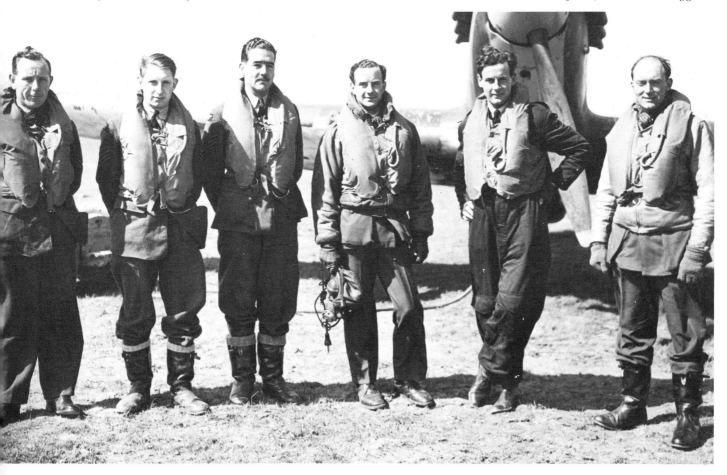

The basic-issue clothing kept a pilot comfortable in flight but provided little protection against such hazards as machine-gun fire. Although combat aeroplanes had armour plating this protected only certain regions of the body, usually the head and chest. Arms and legs were, therefore, in greatest peril from cannon or machine-gun fire. At 18,000 ft over Dorset, Flight Lieutenant Nicholson was rejoining his squadron when an Me110 sneaked on to his tail sending four cannon shells through the Hurricane's cockpit. One shell shattered the perspex canopy, severing his left eyelid, another two hit him in the foot and right leg, the fourth exploded in the auxiliary petrol tank, which caught fire. Taking evasive action he perceived that his attacker had overshot and was now ahead. The instrument panel was beginning to melt in the heat from the fire and both his hands were blistering. Diving he followed the 110, firing his guns until the enemy aircraft was also on fire. Satisfied about its fate he then tried to bale out. He succeeded and spent the next four months in hospital. Nicholson won the only Fighter Command VC of the war for this exploit. Unfortunately no clothing could protect the body from cannon or machine-gun fire.

Fire, fierce, and final, was a pilot's most dreaded enemy. Hurricane and Spitfire aircraft burned rapidly once hit in the right place; a few seconds were all most pilots had for escape, although the clothing a pilot wore would perhaps postpone fatal burns for a vital moment. For this reason pilots were required to wear goggles to protect the eyes; oxygen mask and helmet protected the head and face; the uniform, life-jacket and underwear protected the body, while flying boots and gauntlets (or inner gloves) covered the hands and feet. On one occasion Ginger Lacey, then a Sergeant Pilot with No 501 Squadron, found his aircraft severely damaged when fired on at close quarters by a Heinkel He111. The Hurricane's radiator was shot away and the aircraft set on fire. He baled out. His trousers were burnt off up to the knees and his face was singed. The burns on his face would have been worse had he not been wearing goggles, a precaution many friends had not taken; burnt eyes were fast becoming a fighter pilot's trade mark.

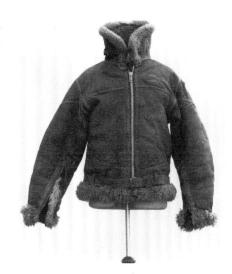

Detail of thermally insulated Flying Jacket as issued.

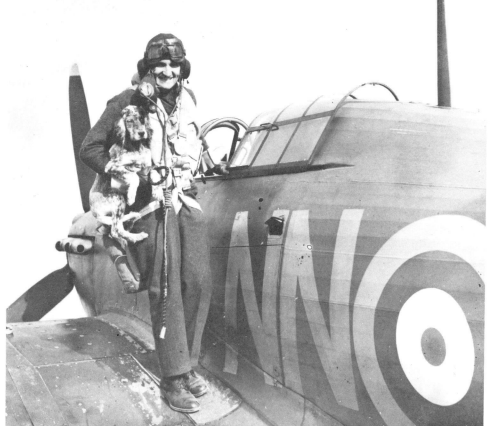

A pilot of No 310 (Czech) Squadron, 1940, in his Type B helmet, D mask and MKIIIA goggles.

Flt. Lt. Johnnie Kent, a famous Battle of Britain fighter pilot standing in front of a 303 Squadron Hurricane. He is wearing a helmet with exposed rubber sockets, MKIV goggles, a Type D oxygen mask and has a yellow painted 1932 pattern life jacket over an Irvin jacket.

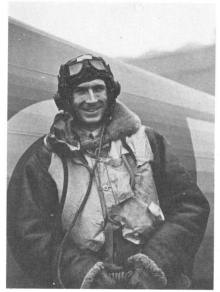

'G' forces

Yet another problem encountered in the skies over Britain in the summer of 1940 was that of 'blackouts'. Violent changes of direction and tight, high 'G' turns at great speed were the cause. With increasing 'G' forces pilots would experience considerable weight increases in their limbs and soft tissues. With positive 'G', blood gets forced away from the brain to the lower parts of the body, resulting in mistiness of vision, 'grey-out', loss of vision and finally 'blackout'. Tests were carried out on a Fairey Battle in spiral dives, and results showed that considerable protection was afforded by adopting a crouching position, while tensing the belly muscles and raising the legs. High and low rudder-bar positions were tried on a Gladiator and later a Spitfire and Hurricane. This test work, carried out by experienced fighter pilots, led to the modification of all fighter aircraft rudder bars. No less than 300 flights were carried out to determine this result, and the young doctor involved blacked out on no fewer than 200 of them.

The death of 'Cobber' Kain, the ace of No 73 Squadron, during the Battle of France at Blois aerodrome on 7 June 1940, pinpoints the dangers of high acceleration. Kain dived his Hurricane inverted towards the aerodrome, pushing through at 350 mph, redding out when blood rushed to his head as 4 'G' negative was applied to his body. Having climbed vertically to 1,500 feet he rolled upright, pushed through again and initiated one, then two, vertical descending rolls. Whether he intended vertical descending rolls is not certain, but it is likely that he was unconscious, as a result of the inrush of blood under pressure to the brain. After two and a half descending rolls the earth intervened, and Cobber Kain died. As a result of the analysis of the incident leading to Kain's death it was at the time felt appropriate that information about 'G' should be supplied to pilots.

It was thought that the Germans who had experimented with a water-filled anti-'G' suit in 1938 were well advanced with this work, however in 1943 when a FW190 landed in the West Country, investigations showed that the pilot was wearing a standard *Luftwaffe* leather flying suit. The Germans had no anti-'G' suit.

"Cobber" Kain, ace pilot of 73 Squadron the Battle of France.

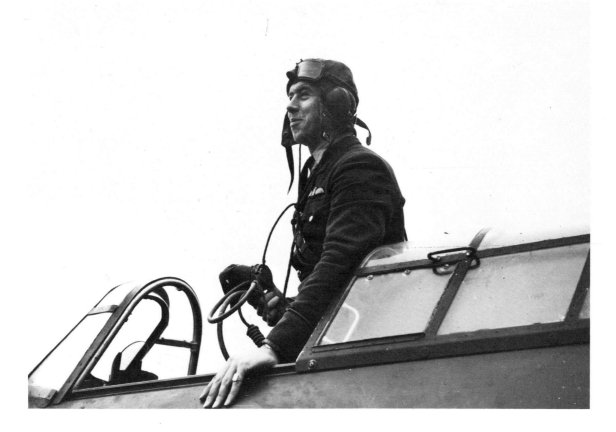

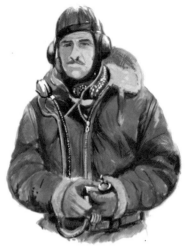

A fighter pilot during the early part of 1940. Wearing a type 'B' helmet fitted with a type 'D' oxygen mask.

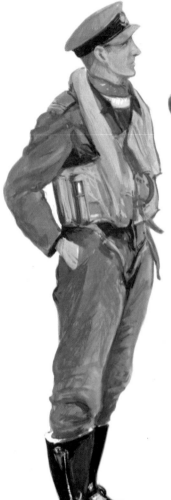

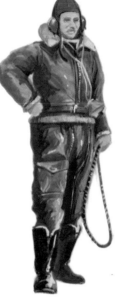

A pilot of a medium bomber in 1940 wearing the complete Irvin Thermally insulated suit and 1936 pattern boots.

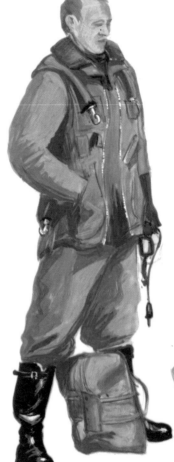

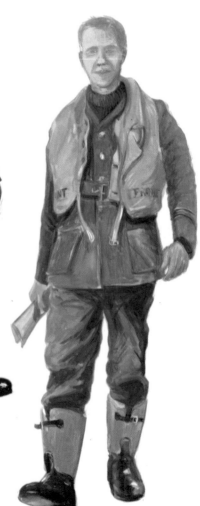

A typical 2nd Tactical Air Force pilot wearing a Mk.I life jacket in a yellow fabric, battle dress and escape boots introduced in 1943.
Pilots were issued with revolvers which were worn in a webbing holster.

A bomber crewman wearing a 1940 pattern flying suit covered by an Irvin harness suit. The boots are 1936 pattern.
Typical of the early war years the crewman would have the type 'B' helmet, but after October 1941 the type 'E' mask and type 'C' helmet became available.

Battle of Britain fighter pilot wearing the 1932 pattern life jacket and 1940 pattern boots.
His helmet would be a type 'B' with type 'D' mask and Mk. IIIa or Mk. IVa or b goggles.
Few fighter pilots wore the Thermally Insulated suits, but many did wear 1930 or 1940 pattern suits. Some chose to wear their pre war black or white prestige overalls. A few retained their squadron badges.

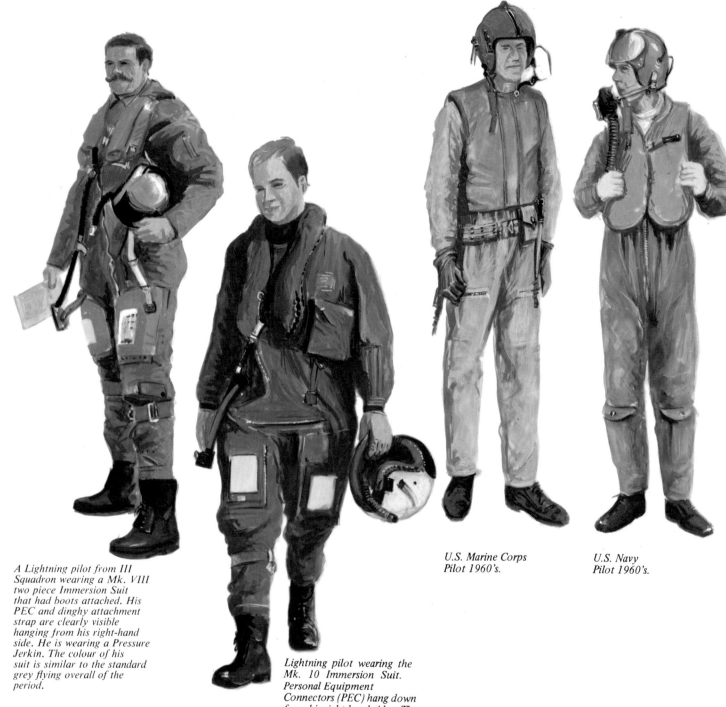

A Lightning pilot from III
Squadron wearing a Mk. VIII
two piece Immersion Suit
that had boots attached. His
PEC and dinghy attachment
strap are clearly visible
hanging from his right-hand
side. He is wearing a Pressure
Jerkin. The colour of his
suit is similar to the standard
grey flying overall of the
period.

Lightning pilot wearing the
Mk. 10 Immersion Suit.
Personal Equipment
Connectors (PEC) hang down
from his right hand sides. The
small strap hanging from his
life preserver on his left
attaches to the dinghy pack
once in the aircraft. Leg
restraint straps which are
attached to the seat, pass
diagonally through buckles
on the garters and prevent
his legs flailing on ejection.

U.S. Marine Corps
Pilot 1960's.

U.S. Navy
Pilot 1960's.

Squadron Leader Franks arrived from Canada in spring 1941 to work at Farnborough. He had already devised a suit of heavy cotton fabric lined with rubber, which fitted the body from the heart level downwards. This suit was filled with water, which, when acted on by 'G', applied pressure on the trunk and lower limbs thus preventing the usual drainage of blood. The suit not only prevented 'blackouts' and reduced pilot fatigue resulting from 'G' forces, but as far as the Navy and Fleet Air Arm were concerned it contained two gallons of drinking water, valuable to men doomed to several days in a rubber dinghy. In 1942 several suits were ordered for trials, and although it showed great advantages, this equipment was heavy and rather cumbersome. The discovery that the Germans did not use anti-'G' suits led to the Frank's suit being dropped.

Professor Cotton in Australia had developed an anti-'G' suit made from rubberised material, known as the 'Pipes of Pan'. Compressed air from a bottle gave graded pressures in different compartments of the suit. A squadron in Darwin had been equipped with this suit, but had abandoned it on account of the heat load on pilots from the impervious rubber. Two of these suits were brought to England by Wing Commander Carr, who did comparative flying trials with the Cotton and Frank's suit. Wing Commander Carr preferred the Cotton suit, which was quite comfortable in a temperate climate. The Americans were the first to introduce anti-'G' suits into service in 1944, and this development encouraged Britain to resume work on them.

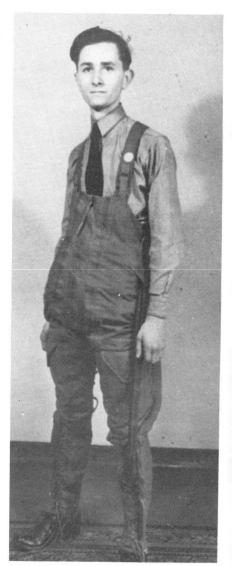

The first American Anti-G suit to be used operationally. The protection given when using this suit was in the region of 2 'G'.

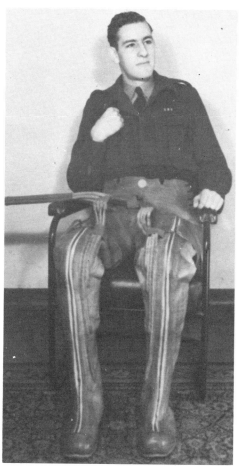

A two piece gradient pressure garment made from rubber and inextensible fabric. It is divided into a series of six overlapping bladders. Protection given was in the order of 3 'G', but the suit was so heavy, clumsy and intolerable under hot conditions, that it was almost unwearable.

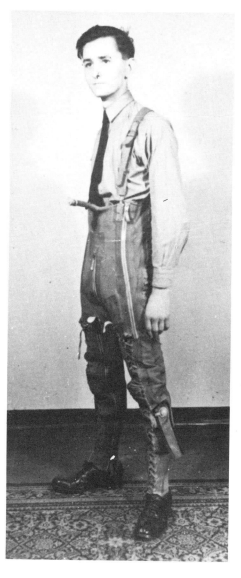

The Franks Mk III suit of 1942. This suit consists of a water bladder encased in an inextensible outer covering.

Service trials in the RAF decided that the suit was undesirable for operational use due to discomfort, maintenance problems, and inability to look behind when wearing the suit. Pilots however reported from 1–2 'G' increase in threshold and lack of fatigue when wearing the suit.

The suit was used operationally by the Fleet Air Arm.

The Mk III suit differed from earlier suits by having the special boots and socks deleted. Seven sizes were available.

Night fighting

By October 1940, the great day-battles had ceased but the 'blitz' was in full swing. Using the cover of darkness, German bombers were striking hard at the cities of Great Britain. Day-fighter squadrons were being used as night fighters, a very hit-and-miss business without the A1 interception radar sets installed in later aircraft. A pilot's eyesight was the prime factor in the night skies. The human eye accommodates itself very well to levels of light and can cope with darkness, given time, a factor not always available to flyers. The retina, the light-sensitive back of the eye, is capable of producing a chemical 'visible purple' which increases its sensitivity. The production of this chemical takes several minutes, but it disperses in only a few seconds. To build up the required sensitivity, red-tinted goggles were issued to all night-fighter aircrews. These were worn on the ground some time before a flight, not only allowing the eyes to develop maximum sensitivity, but also making it possible for the wearer to read and move around in light areas. This equipment was removed when the crews were aboard their aircraft. With Hurricane aircraft the pilot would be treated to the most exciting firework displays from the exhaust pipes, destroying almost immediately his night vision. To prevent this, flat plates were attached to the cowlings above and behind the exhaust pipes to shield the pilot's eyes from the glare. The aircraft types used mainly for night-fighter work were the Blenheim, Defiant, Hurricane, Beaufighter and Mosquito.

The Defiant night-fighter aircraft posed a problem in clothing for the turret-gunner. The small exit from the gun-turret meant that a special parachute suit had to be worn. Made by GQ these parasuits were designed to cover the torso with the parachute harness and parasuit pack built in. The parasuit had no sleeves and had trousers cut short half-way down the thighs. All gunners forced to occupy the turrets in Roc and Defiant aircraft had to be equipped with these suits. Irvin produced a similar torso suit in 1936 known as a harness suit. It did not have an integral parachute and can be distinguished from the GQ suit by having metal clasps, clearly visible on the chest, on which was attached the parachute pack. The Irvin suits were made from a green-coloured fabric.

Pilot and gunner of a 264 Squadro Boulton Paul Defiant that fought in th Battle of Britain. Their clothing is typica The gunner is wearing a Parasuit, a vit piece of equipment for the turret of a Defian These Parasuits were normally grey/green colour.

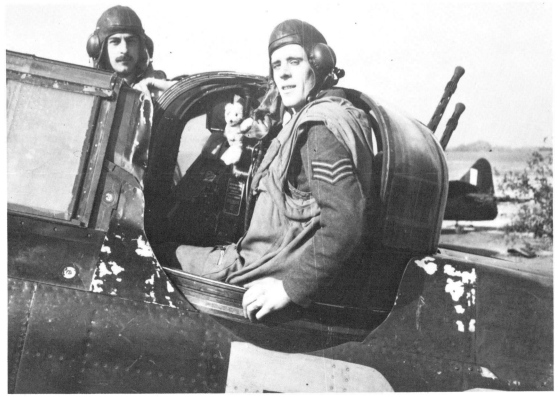

As far as Mosquitos were concerned. an ex-member of No 264 Squadron said that they had such an efficient heating system that the battledress uniform introduced in 1940 worn with standard flying boots were usually quite sufficient to keep aircrews warm, as were the wool-and-rayon vests and drawers issued in 1940. These underclothes were too bulky to wear under the ordinary service-dress uniform so a more roomy blue-grey serge battledress, or 'Suit, Aircrew', to give it the official name, was issued. When flying at night in a Mosquito it was warm enough to wear silk inner gloves rather than the official three pairs of gloves, and these were more sensitive to the controls in the darkness. As well as having a night-fighter role, No 264 Squadron also engaged in attacks on shipping in the Bay of Biscay. The Mosquito was excessively hot in summer on these daylight missions so the crew would frequently fly, with or without permission, in beach attire. The navigator would often carry bottles of water in his map bag; this was good to drink, but even better when poured over oneself.

A night fighter pilot at readiness, wearing night vision glasses. The pilot wears his own white overall and MKI life jacket or Mae West. This was introduced in 1941 and was inflated from a CO_2 bottle rather than by the wearer.

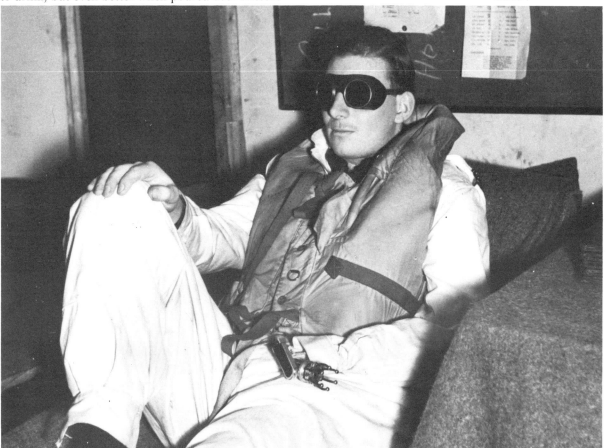

Towards the end of 1941 certain new articles of flying clothing were introduced. The Type 'C' leather helmet superseded the Type 'B'. Unlike the latter it did not have a split at the back with a strap to facilitate ease of fitting, nor did it have zipped leather-covered 'dough-nut' earpieces. It was made from a completely different pattern and was widely used during the war. A new mask, the Type F made of black rubber, was introduced to be worn with the Type C helmet. It was easily recognised by an integral, long, rubber socket into which the convoluted rubber oxygen tube fitted. This was the predecessor of the Type G mask and was the first mask to be used with the economiser system of oxygen delivery. In 1941 a new pattern of flying boot was introduced made of brown suède lined with sheepskin and thirty layers of parachute silk, which provided a splinterproof interlining. These boots were noted for falling off when you baled out, so a modification was made by attaching a leather strap which was buckled round the ankle. This was not completely satisfactory either and aircrew continued to land bootless. In 1941 a new-pattern gauntlet was also introduced.

Other fronts, other clothes

The war against the Axis brought conflict on many fronts. With the invasion of Britain arrested, war flared up in the Mediterranean. Fighter pilots flying in Europe suddenly found themselves in the Western Desert. On the ground it was extremely hot during the day, but in the air it was bitterly cold. Pilots were issued with khaki shorts, trousers and tunics, but as far as flying clothing was concerned the only special issue was that of the Type D fabric helmet, which had a neck protector. This helmet was issued for tropical use in parallel with the Type C helmet which had been introduced in October 1941 for wear in Northern Europe. They were basically similar in design, although the one was made of leather and the other of khaki drill. Very often both types were worn in the desert. The Mk IIIA and Mk IV goggles were used, fitted with tinted lenses. The standard-issue 1940- and 1941-pattern flying boots were a problem, especially in the Far East and Italy where strips became waterlogged after heavy rain and the pilot got his feet wet on the way out to his aircraft. Thus equipped, pilots in the Western Desert, Greece, Crete and Malta prepared for the war in their sector.

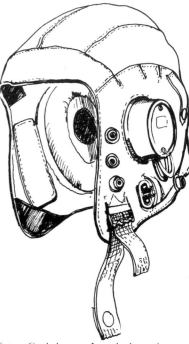

Type C helmet. Issued late in 194 utilising the external wiring harness fron the Type B helmet but being intended to tak the Type E and F masks. Early Type C helmets, Ref 22c 449–452 had leather chi straps. Later versions Ref 22C 877–88 had an integral wiring loom and elasticate chin strap. They were made of dark brow chrome leather, chamois lined. A nava version was also manufactured using 22C/6 zipped earpads as used on the Type B helmet The Type E helmet was made from the sam pattern as the Type C helmet but wa constructed of aertex material. Both th wired and unwired versions had elasticate chin straps. Unwired Ref 22C/744 74 and wired version Ref 22C/973–976. The were intended for use by Coastal Command.

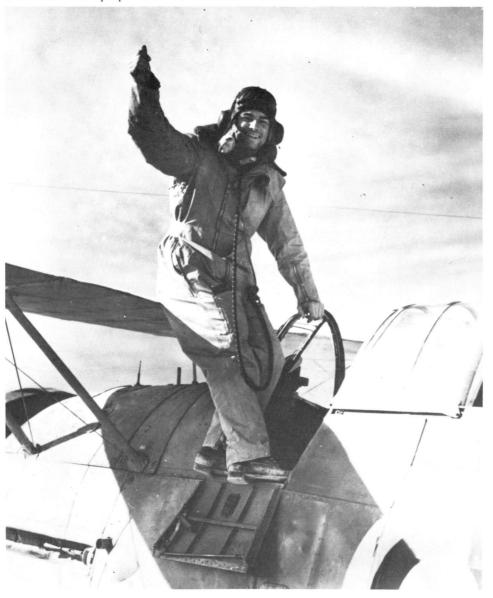

A Gladiator pilot in the Western Desert.

The importance of comfort

In World War II aircrew were able to choose equipment available for issue to suit their requirements, as it was realised that personal comfort made a considerable difference to the successful outcome of combat missions. This was taken to imply that certain personal acquisitions would be overlooked if they supplemented or improved on official issue. One incident of very unofficial dress was noted in the desert when Wing Commander Jackie Darwin took command of 224 Wing. He was a keen sportsman and thought hunting the desert fox a good idea. Squadron members crowded into jeeps which drove into the desert and were driven round until a fox was sighted. The Wing mascot, a dog called 'Rommel', was then launched from a moving jeep in pursuit of the fox. However, he usually took off in the opposite direction and the hunt would end in attempting to recapture him. Darwin had with him his hunting outfit which he wore on such occasions. Once while in mid-hunt the Wing was brought to immediate readiness and Wing Commander Darwin, dressed for the kill, had to get airborne in his Hurricane. Later, dodging flak, he caught the ground with his propeller and had to make a forced landing. A patrolling armoured car rescued him and he was eventually taken to an army mess where the CO greeted him with, 'This is the first time I've seen an RAF officer properly dressed.'

Group of pilots from a Gladiator squadron in the Middle East displaying an interesting collection of equipment; 1932 Pattern life jackets in grey/green, khaki tropical kit, 1936 Pattern boots, desert boots, a white and a khaki lightweight flying overalls and MKII goggles with tinted lenses. Their helmets all appear to be Type B with Type D masks.

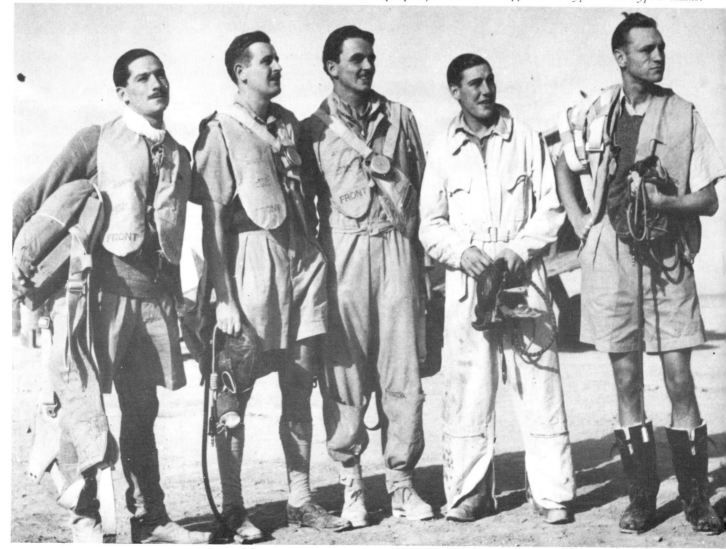

Mr John Brooks, recently retired as a senior captain in British Airways, wrote this fascinating account of the different equipment he wore as a fighter pilot in Northern Europe and the Mediterranean:

After completing my basic square-bashing, I was posted to ITW (Initial Training Wing) at Cambridge. Here *all* future pilots were given instructions into the mysteries of Navigation, Gunnery, Met., Air Force law etc. We were also given our flying kit for our Tiger Moth training. This consisted of:

1 Light green Sidcot 1940 pattern – with a fur collar and zips everywhere.
2 One pair of shiny leather boots, fleecy lined. 1936 pattern.
3 The three pairs of gloves – silk, wool and leather gauntlets (but without fire protection paint on them, this came later).
4 Leather helmet with the zip ear covers – plus goggles.
5 Gosport tubes (for Tiger Moths).
6 A number of combination sets of fine wool which I immediately sent to my father for his fire-watching duties.

After passing out at Cambridge (I was at Downing) my course was sent to Prestwick for Tiger Moth training (or as we called them – 'Tigerschmitts'). Then on to Montrose from Prestwick for Master 1 flying.

At Montrose we flew about twenty-five hours on the Master 1s. Still no radio so we stuck to our Gosports. We also flew Hurricanes if we were successful in passing out. We were then promoted to Sgt-Pilot at the same time as we got our Wings. There was no parade or suchlike 'bull'. We were simply told to sew Sgt stripes and Wings on the LAC uniform and report to the Sgts' mess.

Next step was Hurricane OTU (Operational Training Unit). Here we at last got our oxygen mask plus radio earphones and mic. We also got issued with Irvin jacket and trousers, and a couple of Navy-type white pullovers.

I never wore the Irvin clobber except one occasion when I was doing patrols at night over London. It was winter and very cold, and since we had to stay up for

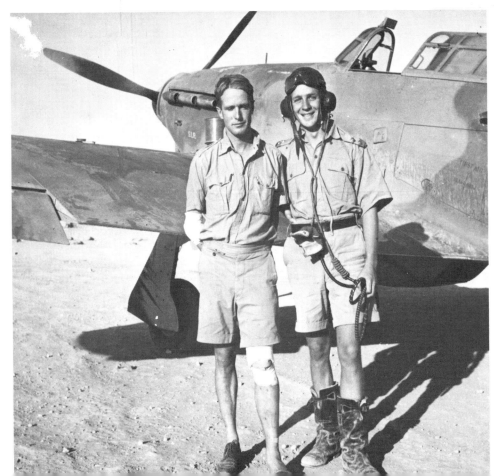

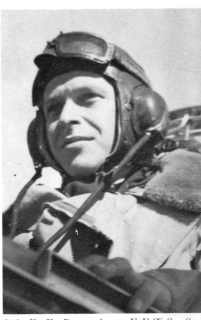

Desert Hurricane pilots in 1941.

Cpl. F. E. Dymond, 32 E.F.T.S., Swi[ft] Current, Canada, in his Tiger Mo[th] wearing MKIIIA goggles, Type B helme[t] 1940 Pattern Suit and Gosport Tube[s] otherwise known as "Profanity Strainers".

a couple of hours, you got frozen. They were too bulky to wear in a fighter, but I know that the Bomber boys used them all the time over Europe.

So apart from our normal clothing and uniforms packed in a white canvas kit bag, we were lumbered with all this extra flying kit. At the Hurricane OTU we completed about twenty-five hours on type–gunnery, formation flying, aerobatics, low flying, cross country, etc, and then it was off to a squadron.

I went to 607 Squadron (County of Durham). It was apparently a custom for the Auxiliary Squadron Officers to have red lining to their overcoats; at least, so I was informed. This did not apply to other ranks.

1941–2

It was whilst I was on this squadron that I was issued with a parachute and Mae West. These were personal issue, and they became yours for all time. The parachute was fitted to you like a suit, made nice and comfy. The straps that went between the legs were most important and made to fit quite tightly.

The parachute opened with such a jerk that loose straps could do you an injury–you'd end up by singing soprano. This type of chute fitted into the bucket seat of fighters; we carried no dinghy as yet–only a rubber cushion between our rears and the parachute.

We were also given a revolver (what for, I can't imagine) and a commando knife. Later, each pilot was given various escape aids as the backroom boys thought them up. Since we were now operating over France nearly every day during the 'shooting season', it was considered prudent to take great notice of all these gadgets.

There were magnetic fly-buttons, the compass in the collar stud, the dirty oily handkerchief which was really a map of France. There were also 'iron-ration' packs with all sorts of goodies inside–and of course, a great wad of French and German money. Unfortunately this had to be handed back to the Spy (Intelligence Office) after each trip.

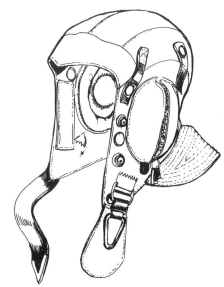

Type D helmet. Made from exactly the same pattern as the Type C but was made of khaki twill material. Because it was intended for tropical wear it has a neck protector attached to the back. The early Type D helmet was unwired and had the rubberised microphone sockets stitched to the outside as opposed to being fitted from the inside. These also had leather chin straps. Ref 22C/581–584. The later type D, Ref 22C/969–972, was wired and featured the elasticated chin strap. The naval version of the Type D was fitted with 22C/66 zipped earpads.

A Flying Training School, probably in Rhodesia.

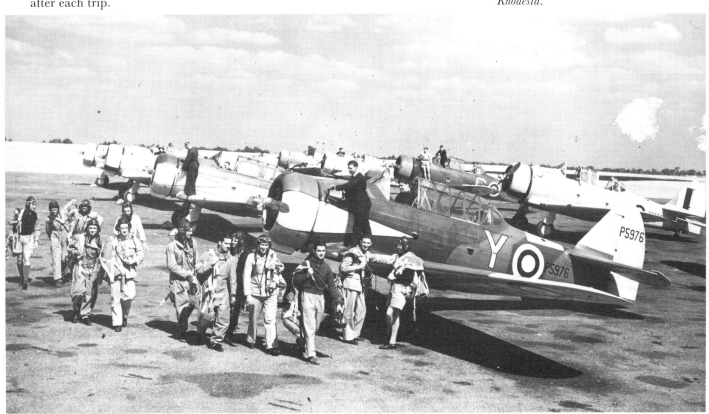

Then of course we had a civilian jacket and beret, but this was very hush-hush for obvious reasons.

So to the dressing up – which was done in the flight hut on the airfield and went something like this.

We usually had our blue battledress with a navy pullover (this superseded the Frock White). We had nowhere to put the collar-stud compass until one bright boy told us, but it was considered too uncomfortable. We tucked our trousers into the flying boots, with long socks sent to us by the girls in the Gas Board Offices in Sandwich, God bless 'em.

It was usual to wear your civilian jacket under your battledress blouse, with the beret tucked inside. Next came the Mae West, and again tucked inside this were the iron rations and money pack. Down the boots were pushed a map, commando knife and revolver. You were now pretty well loaded. Staggering awkwardly out to your Hurricane, you put on your parachute and climbed in, usually being pushed from behind by one of the ground crew. Once strapped in, you adjusted your seat and rudder pedals, made certain your rear-seeing mirror was OK, then put on your helmet, plugging in the oxygen and radio. Lastly you put on the three pairs of gloves. You were now ready for the fray. (Very awkward if now you wanted to spend a penny – it was a good plan to do it before 'kitting up').

As a squadron we normally flew in close formation, but once over the other side you opened up in what was termed battle formation. It was my personal drill to turn on my reflector sight and gun button to 'fire'. I also used to drop my seat a notch or two – not that this did any good but it made me feel safer. I then lowered my goggles so that the face was now completely covered.

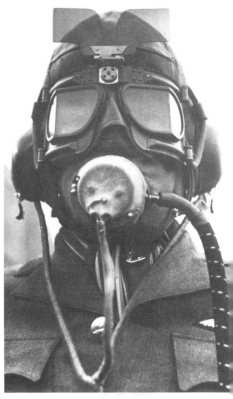

A Royal Canadian Air Force fighter pilot in his Type B helmet, Type D mask and MKIVA goggles.

1942

I was sent overseas towards the end of 1942, and was given the kit to go there. KD shorts and shirts, also long trousers, mosquito boots and net. And since I was now commissioned, I had to carry all the officers' clobber and what was known as a 'camp kit'. This was a sort of large canvas sack into which you put sheets and blankets to make a bed. Rather like a sleeping bag. This was put on a concertina trestle arrangement. A canvas wash basin and chair completed the ensemble. It weighed a ton. Of course, it was necessary to take our parachute in its nice neat bag. It was so easy to lose the odd item of kit especially as we were travelling about so much.

The Americans were so entranced with our battledress that they tended to wear it themselves. The squadron I was attached to in Italy (249) came under US control and so we were told that we were entitled to US facilities, which included kitting out at their expense. I should explain that during the North African and Italian campaigns we RAF (including all the other Air Forces of the Empire) wore khaki. The only difference was our blue hats and the blue stripes of rank.

The US supplied us with battledress of similar design to the British but was altogether much superior in every way. For one thing, it was made of a very soft woollen cloth, like a fine Melton – albeit slightly darker colour than our khaki. The shirts, very dark, also were out of this world, beautifully made, and they never seem to wear out. I was still wearing one up to last year, that is some thirty years after they were issued to me. Other things like underwear were all of the same standard – and we got them all free.

In fact, the US gave our Wing (three squadrons) our own light bomber (a Mitchell) modified for leave purposes. They were most generous in every way and I have a soft spot for the Yanks. (I won't go into the treatment I got from our other ally.)

Another thing the US supplied us with were very nice woollen blankets, also the same dark khaki colour, with a big US stamped in the middle. I had one made into an overcoat later on, after the war was over, and I believe my mother still has one at home.

All these 'gifts' from the US were given to *all* ranks, not just officers and NCOs. I liked that.

The mud in Italy was often impossible. Even to walk was difficult and as for flying, we often couldn't move our aircraft. Most of the lads bought brown dispatch-riders' boots—long lace-up affairs, and then had an extra sole made of Me109 tyre, put on. This was done by itinerant Italian shoemakers who were always around in camp. Sort of camp-followers, along with the ubiquitous Italian washer-women.

As officers, we could get replacement clothing from the local officers' shop. We had to pay, naturally, but it was such a nominal sum and being in the 'field', we had nothing else to spend our pay on. The officers' shop was usually at one of the main rear bases. In the beginning of the Sicilian Campaign it was on Malta with another in Tunis. I believe they were supplied from Cairo. Later as we moved forward, the shop was at Catania, then Naples and later Rome.

Although we all wore some form of khaki battledress, the pilots still had their own uniforms. There was the usual mixture of air forces in 249 Squadron—this became common later on in the war. There were South Africans who had South African Army ranks and uniforms, Canadians, Aussies, NZ, Poles, French, etc. On one occasion, the American Commander (a Major-Gen) of the heavy bomber group, which it was our job to escort, invited our Spitfire Wing Officers for a drink (actually a wing-ding of a party). These US airmen had been used to seeing us in our khaki, so that when we turned up in our best uniforms they were utterly astounded to see so many different colours and hues, apart from the shapes. In fact one wisecracker said we only needed a *Luftwaffe* uniform to make up the set.

Since there was a war on, nobody worried about proper dress. We seemed to just put on what was available, including some items 'won' from the enemy.

The result was that we ended up with an odd assortment of clothing, Navy, Army, Air Force, plus US, *Luftwaffe* and *Regia Aeronautica* (including the odd aeroplane).

I believe the local Forces newspaper in the Med. area, the Eighth Army News, ran a comic strip cartoon called 'The Three Types'. These were typical and portray the situation perfectly.

One thing we did was to share out the kit of any of our lads who got themselves shot down. This may appear to be rather macabre, but we knew that it would be rifled anyway at the rear base, so it was better to know that your friends had it. Of course personal effects, such as letters, etc were sent separately to the next of kin—together with log book, photos and anything of value.

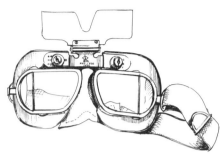

Goggles MK VII. They featured a very heavy brass frame painted ultramarine blue as well as split safety lenses and a pull-down polarised screen.

1944–5

After I left Italy, just south of the Po Valley, I went to Cairo and became a gunnery instructor. This was in the Canal Zone.

Then after the war ended I went to Transport Command operating all over the world. I and my crew were sometimes away from our base in Alamarza, Cairo, for as long as six or seven weeks, which meant we became rather like gypsies, carrying all our possessions with us in our beloved Dakota. It became like our home.

Most of the time I wore bush jackets and shorts, long khaki socks and I never seemed to be out of them. I still prefer the desert boot than anything else.

1946

I was eventually posted home in 1946—after something like four years overseas. I embarked from Port Said in charge of 400 Air-Force personnel, on a very nice boat. This took us to Marseilles where we boarded a train to Calais. Then on another boat to Dover, train to somewhere in the Midlands, Cardington I think. And I didn't lose one of my 400 chaps.

Here we were all demobbed after medicals etc. It was like joining up in reverse.

Then we were led around a huge warehouse where you chose your civvy gear—suit, hat, mac, shoes and shirts.

We also handed in any kit we didn't want, including guns, ammo and sun-dried bric-à-brac which had accumulated over the years.

And that was that.

The Luftwaffe

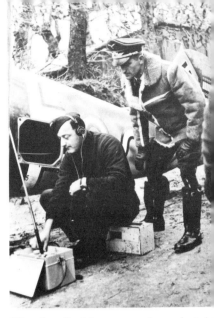

If the sky could be so inhospitable for the RAF, it is reasonable to suppose that the *Luftwaffe* shared the same problems. However, since 1933 the Germans had put a lot of effort into the medical aspects of flying. By the start of World War II the *Luftwaffe* had a series of flying clothing outfits which supplied all their needs, and they had experimented with 'G' suits and pressure suits, although these were not issued to aircrew. Their basic equipment consisted of black suède, sheepskin-lined, calf-length flying boots with zips: three types of flying overall: the lightweight summer type in khaki cotton material issued to all aircrew but usually worn by bomber and reconnaissance aircraft crews; the 'Bavarian', a blue-grey velvet overall with a dark brown fur collar which, unlike the lightweight summer overall, did not normally have rank badges displayed on it. The third type was the brown leather winter suit which was belted at the waist, had a blue velvet collar and was lined. A light blue cotton overall was also available with electrically heated gloves and socks. Fighter pilots were allowed black leather flying jackets, popularly worn over their *Luftwaffe* uniform in preference to flying overalls.

The Germans did not incorporate microphones in their oxygen masks, all helmets had throat microphones attached. There were three basic helmet types available: the summer helmet, made from chocolate brown Aertex cotton material; the winter helmet in leather to the same pattern; and the cold weather helmet which was again to the same pattern but fleece lined. Helmets were issued in an unwired condition, but were later fitted with Siemens telephones, a standard and very neat design, produced in Bakelite. Grooves were moulded on the outside face of each telephone to accommodate goggle straps, eliminating the need for strap buckles and press-studs, so familiar on RAF helmets. Leitz, the famous optical firm, produced darkened shatter-proof goggles for purchase to the standard *Luftwaffe* issue.

The pilot of a Me 109, wearing a sheepsk coat watches as radio tests are carried ou Battle of Britain period.

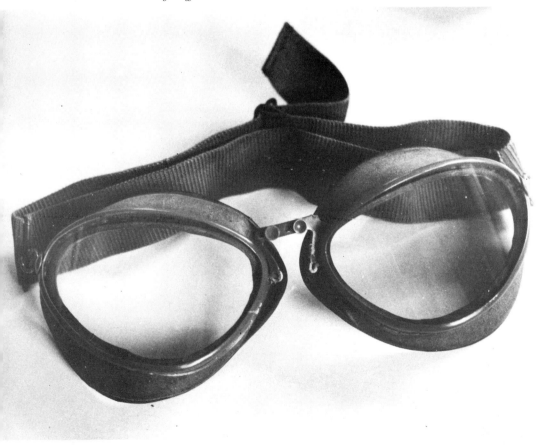

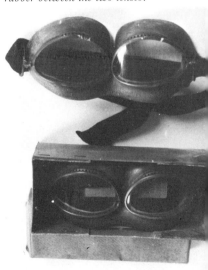

Standard issue German goggles of Wor War II. Both used the same lenses an had interchangeable, clear or tinted lense The principal difference was that one had adjustable bridge whereas the other had th lenses set in a rubber mask. Adjustment to t latter could be made by piercing holes in t rubber between the two lenses.

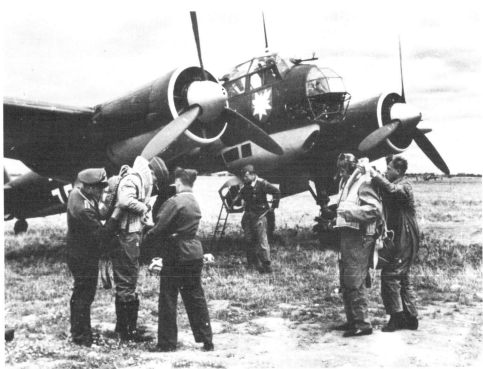

In France, during the Battle of Britain, a Ju 88 crew make ready.

In 1937, using He111 and Do17 bombers, the Germans worked on the problem of oxygen supply for aircrew. The equipment used provided adequate protection to altitudes of 26,200ft. The rule was that oxygen should always be used above 13,000ft, and on long flights above 8,200ft. Until 1936 a constant-flow oxygen system was available, controlled by the user. After 1936 the Auer A-824 demand regulator was developed. This device allowed oxygen to be conserved, and was the first of such systems to be used in quantity. The 10-38 demand regulator, operated by an aneroid capsule, automatically adjusted the oxygen flow in relation to the altitude, and at 26,000ft a delivery of 100 per cent was attained. This regulator came into use in 1937. Development was rapid and by 1939 a 10-137 regulator would supply oxygen under pressure to allow adequate delivery to aircrew at altitudes above 26,200ft. This sytem was standard on all *Luftwaffe* aircraft until the end of the war.

The crew of a Heinkel 111 bomber wearing fawn lightweight summer suits, standard Kapok-filled life jackets and summer and winter helmets. The oxygen masks and tubes hang from the life jackets. In use the mask was attached over the sides and crown of the helmet with straps.

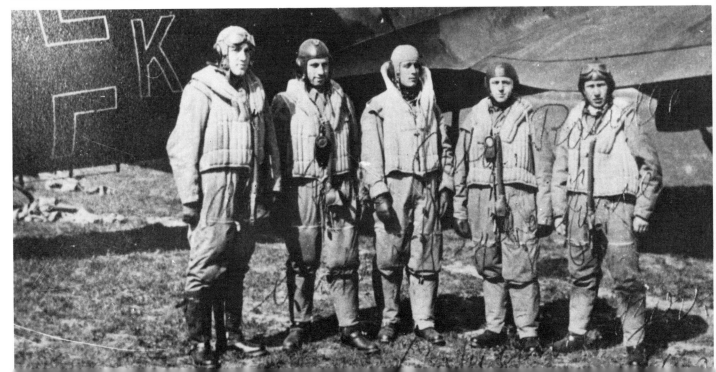

Side by side with their work on regulators, the Germans led the field in oxygen mask design. In 1934 a quick-disconnect mask was developed by Drägerwerke. Researchers found that freezing of the masks was difficult to overcome, heated oxygen was found to be harmful, and so electrically heated masks were tried. In 1939 a mask was developed in which the warmth of exhaled air prevented the mask from freezing. This item remained standard, although the *Luftwaffe* planned to adopt a copy of the American A-10-A oxygen mask, which did not rip from the face when a pilot had to bale out. Because of the collapse of German war production the 1944 A-10-A copy did not go into production. German oxygen masks were produced in black rubber, the oxygen tube suspended from a valve in the centre. The mask covered the nose and mouth and was small by comparison with the Types 'G' and 'H' masks used by the Allies since it did not contain a microphone.

I have not seen any evidence of German buoyancy or survival suits but it is possible these were available; however, there seems to have been two basic types of life-jacket. One, favoured by bomber and transport aircraft crews, was made from natural-coloured fabric with kapok-padded cells disposed vertically down the jacket. This garment circled the neck and was secured around the wearer's torso. The second type, generally used by the occupants of fighter aircraft, who had less room in their cockpits, was made of rubber, with a small CO_2 bottle to inflate it. The rubber was a naples rather than chrome yellow in colour.

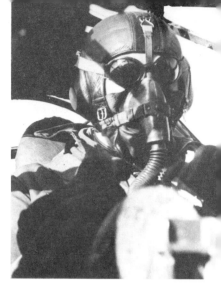

The pilot of a HeIII wears a brown leather helmet, Nitsche Gunter goggles and as the photograph shows, an oxygen mask and its attachments. Throat microphones were standard.

The crew of a Focke Wolf 200 Condor prepare for a flight.

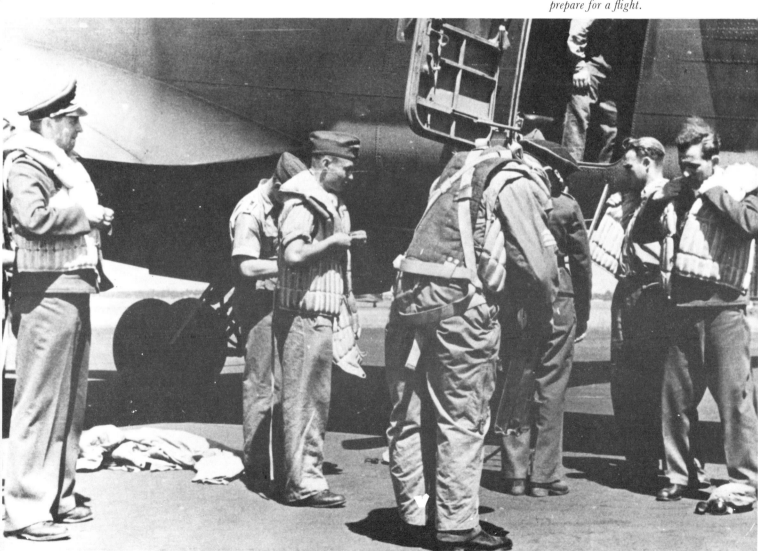

When the American daylight bomber offensive really got under way in 1943, the *Luftwaffe* was desperately trying just about every imaginable way of getting interceptor aircraft produced and into the fight. One aircraft developed to meet this threat was the critical Me163 Komet rocket fighter. The machine had a terrific rate of climb which enabled it to get above the bomber formations quickly. With the fuel exhausted the machine would dive at a selected target, despatch its armament and glide back to base. The tremendous thrust of these machines was achieved by mixing T-stoff, forty-eight per cent concentrated hydrogen peroxide and a mixture of hydro-carbon compounds, with C-stoff which was thirty per cent hydrazine hydrate solution in methyl alcohol: a well-nigh lethal mixture if it got anywhere near the pilot. The following extract from *Rocket Fighter* by Mano Ziegler illustrates some of the problems encountered by the Me163 pilots:

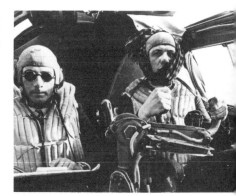

Pilot and navigator of a He 111.

> It could happen that our oxygen system malfunctioned or received damage from enemy fire, and if we were unable to recognize altitude symptoms immediately we would have virtually no chance of returning to earth alive. We were told that immediately we experienced such symptoms it was our duty to put the nose of the fighter down and dive for the safety of the 4,000-metre line. This all applied, of course, to any aircraft flying at extreme altitudes, but a climb to altitude taking perhaps thirty minutes in an orthodox fighter was an affair of hardly more than a minute in a rocket-driven fighter. With a sinking feeling in the pit of my stomach, I made way for the next batch of pressure-chamber guinea-pigs and, together with Fritz and Herbert, made my way to the stores to collect the 'powered egg' pilot's outfit. This included all the usual accessories, such as fur-lined boots, flying helmet with built-in headphones, R/T connection leads, parachute pack, flying gloves, etcetera, but to this pile was added a combination smock manufactured of allegedly acid-proof material! Fritz commented, seeing the question that I was about to ask, 'When the T-stoff flows into your pants instead of finding its way into the combustion chamber you burn up like a firework, and this will slow down the process!' 'How come?' I asked. 'Well, it sometimes happens that a feedline develops a leak or a fuel tank explodes!' he replied. I needed no further explanation!

The crewman of a Dornier wearing a steel helmet over a summer weight helmet. The life jacket is a fawn coloured inflatable more commonly worn in fighter aircraft.

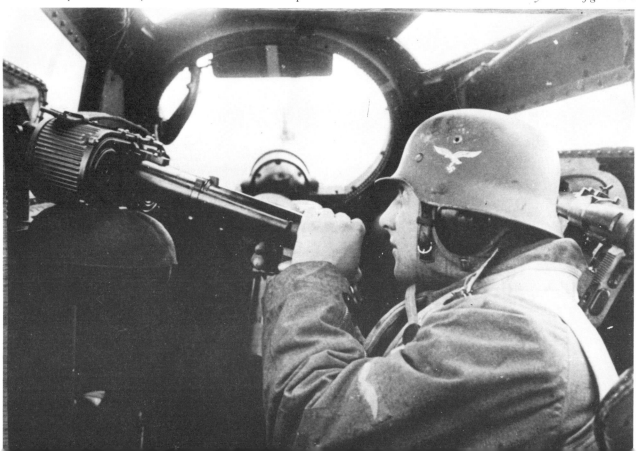

Jets on the horizon

Throughout the course of World War II fighter pilots saw very few changes in their basic equipment. It was inevitable that with the increasing demand for pilots the clothing items had to be mass produced; the result was that helmets, jackets, masks, gloves, boots and overalls remained standard even though they would be worn by pilots in Greece, Malta, Cyprus, Italy, on fighter sweeps over Northern Europe, on escort duties or while flying against the Japanese in Burma.

The performance of most World War II fighter aircraft represented great technical advances, but these brought few changes to the flying clothing issued. Even when RAF Bomber Command operated large daylight raids in conjunction with the United States Army Air Force, and fighter pilots had to offer themselves for long escort duties, no extras were offered for the pilots' comfort. The sole relief for tired limbs and sore bottoms was to squirm around as much as possible. The only innovations of any significance to RAF war-time fighter pilots were the more comfortable 1940-pattern flying suit, the economiser system of oxygen delivery which was introduced at the end of 1941 along with the Type C helmet and Type F and later the G mask, and the CO_2 inflating life-jacket.

Air Vice Marshal Bouchier talking pilots of the County of Durham Auxilia Squadron, August 1945, in South Ea Asia.
USAAF fighter pilots wearing both Briti and American helmets.

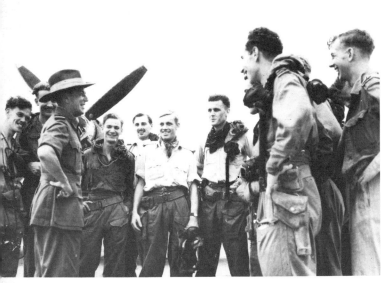
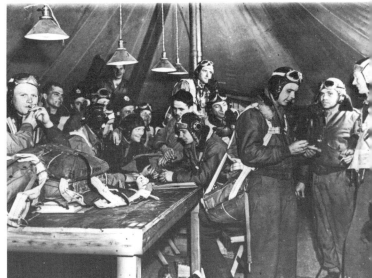

It was not until the advent of jet aircraft and ejector seats that more highly specialised flying clothing was introduced, although no particular clothing was introduced to accompany the Meteor, Britain's first jet fighter, into service in 1944. Nor were pilots of jet aircraft to appear as strange as the following tale depicts.

Late in 1942 a flight of USAAF P38 Lightnings was leisurely cruising on a training mission in the vicinity of Muroc Dry Lake, California, when their astonished pilots found themselves accompanied by a weird apparition – a propellerless aircraft from the cockpit of which a gorilla grimaced at them. What was worse, the gorilla was wearing a black derby hat and smoking a cigar! This fantastic interloper formated briefly with the Lightnings and then dived away to be rapidly lost to sight, while some badly shaken trainee fighter pilots returned to their base and to the derision that inevitably greeted their story. Some time was to elapse before they were to learn that they had been victims of a hoax perpetrated by a Bell test pilot, Jack Woolams. Wearing a gorilla Hallowe'en mask, Woolams had been flying the first American jet aircraft, the highly secret XP-59A Airacomet.

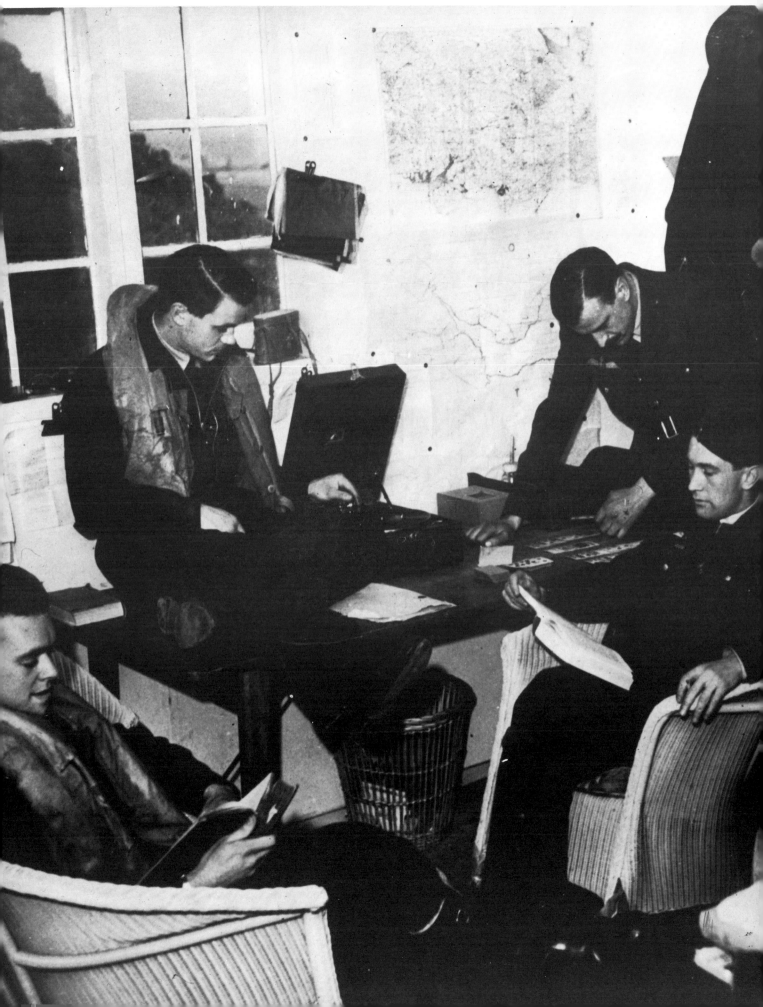

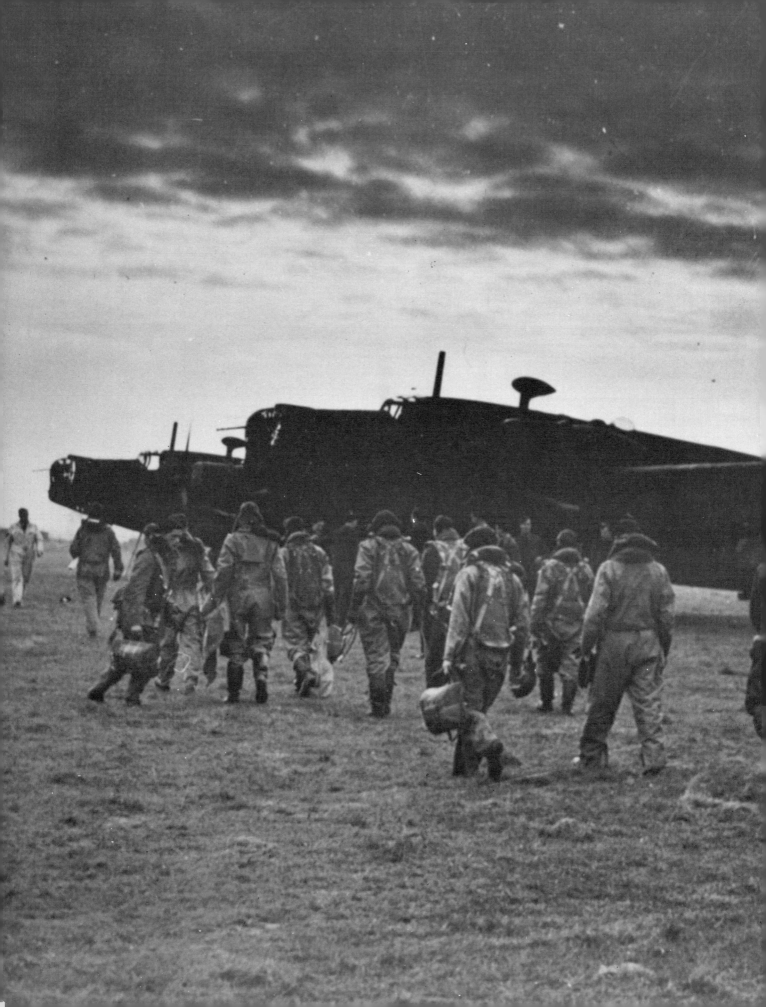

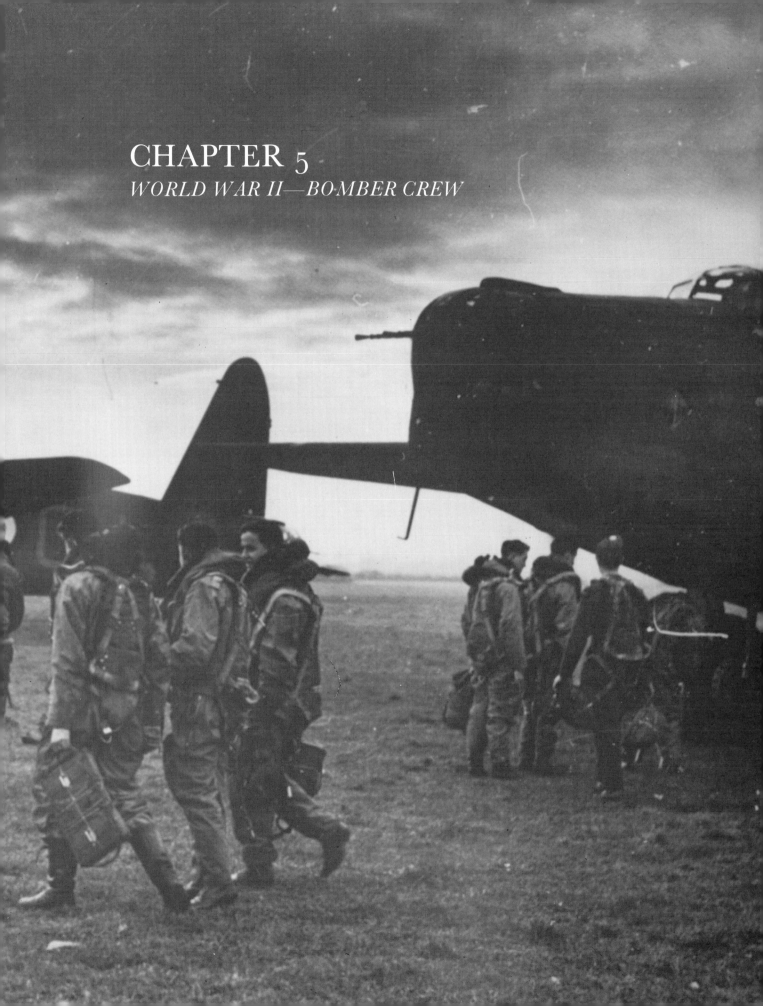

CHAPTER 5
WORLD WAR II—BOMBER CREW

While RAF fighters intercepted bombers and duelled with enemy fighters, another great Command struggled night after night over Germany: Bomber Command, which was to grow between 1939 and 1945 into a massive operational machine. Unlike their fighter-pilot colleagues, the crew of bomber aircraft had to sustain their flights for five, six or more hours, and to learn to put up with many hazards. Cold was an ever-present problem. The night sky did not offer much comfort, and although bomber aircraft were heated, the equipment was not always efficient and did not serve all occupied parts of the machine. Flak, enemy night fighters, system failures, weather changes, fire, communications failure, oxygen failure and fatigue were other crosses bomber crewmen had to bear philosophically.

As a result of the expansion programmes started in 1936, Bomber Command had Wellington, Whitley and Hampden aircraft as heavy types, with Blenheim and Battle aircraft as medium bombers by the time war broke out. The two types of medium machine were sent in small numbers to France in 1939 and were massacred in daylight raids on strategic targets. As a result Battles were withdrawn from service, but Blenheims remained in service until 1943.

Blenheim crews wearing Irvin thermal insulated suits. The person on the right wearing the newly introduced 1940 Patte boots.

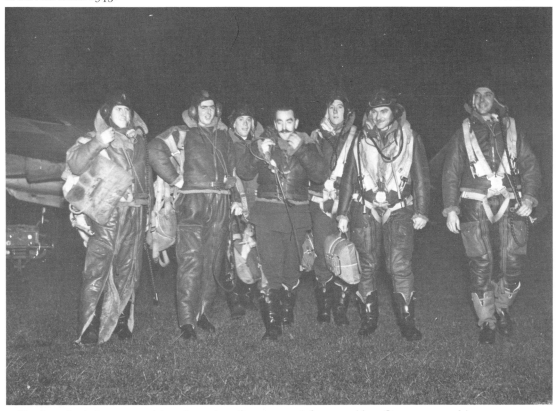

During the 'phoney war' bomber aircraft were used for attacking German warships, dropping propaganda leaflets and mine-laying, but when the Germans overran the Low Countries and France in May and June 1940, Bomber Command was placed in an offensive role and was tasked to delay and weaken the German advance by destroying enemy lines of communications and supply. Strategic bridges, railway junctions, marshalling yards and oil dumps in Western Germany and enemy-occupied territory were repeatedly bombed. But many of these attacks, especially by night, were not successful. In 1940 only one-third of raiding aircraft managed to place their bombs within a five-mile radius of an intended target. Even a large city was difficult to locate by night for at this stage of the war there were few navigational aids. Photographic equipment installed in bomber aircraft made it abundantly clear that accurate bombing was rare. It is interesting to note that the Air Ministry gave the job of organising the Photographic Reconnaissance Unit (PRU) at Heston to Sidney Cotton, the Australian who gave his name to the Sidcot Suit.

Bombers on the warpath

The bombing offensive was intensified in the autumn of 1940 and during 1941. The Battle of Britain had been fought and won, thus more emphasis could be placed on attack than on defence. Hundreds of heavy aircraft droned their way through the unknown night skies to rain bombs on the enemy. Daylight raids had been largely abandoned as they had resulted in heavy losses.

The situation improved when Sir Arthur Harris became Commander-in-Chief of Bomber Command on 22 February 1942. Harris had the leadership really to make the Command work, using heavy bombers such as the recently introduced Stirling, Halifax and Lancaster to destroy the enemy's manufacturing capabilities and their morale by saturation bombing. On the night of 30–31 May 1942 he launched the first 'thousand-bomber' raid against Cologne. The raid was a success, with a reduction in the loss of crews and machines. The incendiary area bombing led to the policy of precision night bombing being quietly shelved, although the US Eighth Air Force, which arrived in Britain in 1942, was attempting daylight precision bombing from their high-flying B-17s. Radio navigation aids like 'OBOE' and 'GEE' made the location of targets easier, and a later device H$_2$S, enabled crews to pinpoint areas of a city through cloud.

To aid the great armadas of heavy bombers to unload their bombs effectively at night a special force was created, the famous Pathfinders. Their job was to fly ahead of the main force, and accurately to locate and mark targets. The crews assigned to these missions were considered the best in the Command. Many crews in the Pathfinder Force used the Mosquito, when it became available, an aircraft whose speed, war load and small operating crew made it perhaps the most efficient bomber of the war. Raids were carried out by Bomber Command, razing great cities like Hamburg, Munich and Dresden to charred rubble. This destructive success owed much to the skilled incendiary marking by the Pathfinders. So effective was this target pinpointing, that bombs would land within 1,000 yards of their intended target.

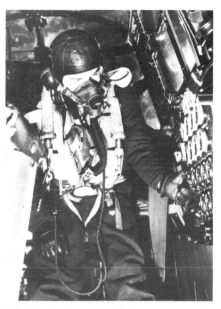

The Flight Engineer at his instrument panel, showing the severe space limitations inside a Lancaster. He is wearing the Type B helmet with special attachments to take the Type G mask. The metal plates above the ear pieces are for holding MKIV goggles.

Paratroopers marching out to board a Whitley. Note the distinctive helmet design.

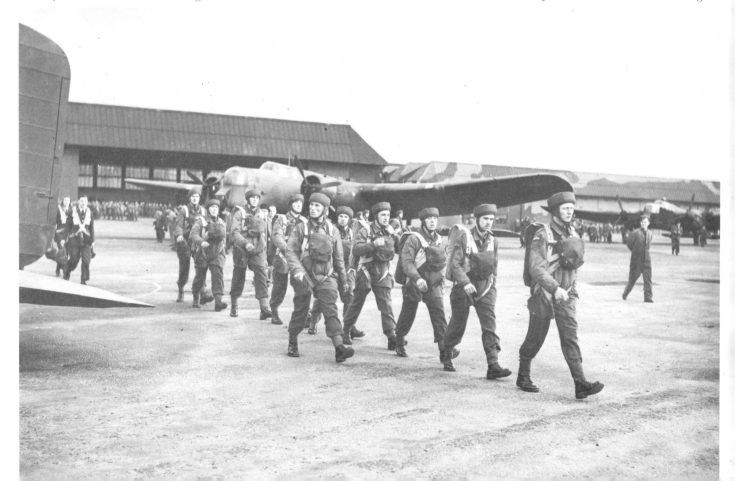

The Germans were not passive about the offensive and operated a complex night-fighter network, controlled by radar, and supplemented by 'NAXOS' equipment which allowed a night fighter to get within visual range of its target. Because America was unable to supply ·5 cannons for defence, heavy bombers were equipped with ·303 machine-guns which had a limited effective range. This meant that cannon-equipped German night fighters could blow bombers out of the sky without even getting within range of the bombers' defensive armament. The Germans also concentrated a great deal of their war effort on producing and manning anti-aircraft guns.

To confuse German radar plots aircraft of 100 Group were equipped with jamming devices. The crews of these aircraft, often Stirlings, had sometimes to supply diversionary imitations for two separate raids in one night. They were able to sustain long hours in the air by having no bomb load, thus being able to carry extra fuel. These aircraft also carried out solo missions with electronic engineers on board, whose job it was to study new advances in German radar and invent new jamming devices.

Again, the cold

The bomber crew's main problem was that of cold. The cockpit heating system may have been effective but rarely was any heat provided in other parts of the aircraft. The crew often had to man their positions for six or more hours while the aircraft ploughed its way through the bitter night sky. They had little chance to move around, and cold soon set in.

A Whitley crew demonstrate the variety and types of clothing used in bombers in the early years of the war.

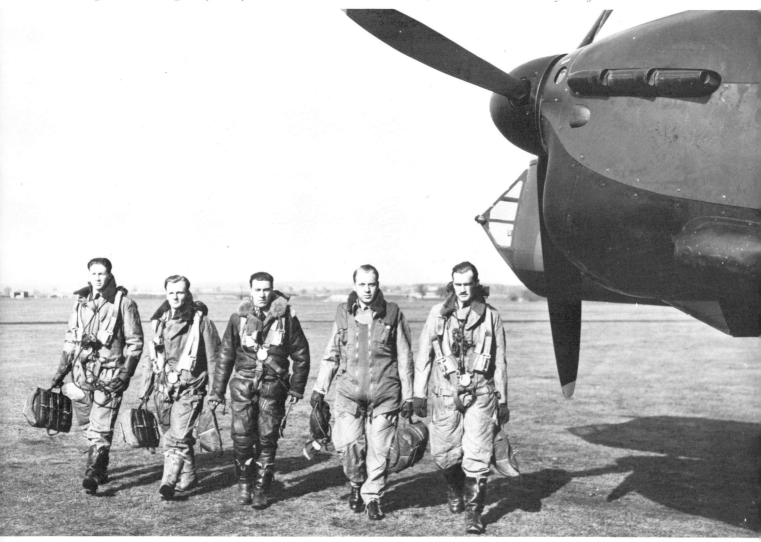

The standard equipment for all crews consisted of combination underwear (some men used their girl friends' silk stockings as well) a uniform, many pairs of woollen socks, a Frock White pullover, an inner quilted lining, an outer 1930- or 1940-pattern overall, electrically heated moccasins and gloves, silk gloves, mittens and leather gauntlets as well as Type B or C helmet. The 1941-pattern flying boot had fairly wide ankles and could therefore comfortably accommodate the electrically heated moccasins. The 1943-pattern black suède boot was not so popular as the shoe part was a tighter fit. However, this boot was particularly useful if for one reason or another you found yourself in enemy territory, since a small knife was incorporated in the strap of the boot which was used to cut off the boot uppers, leaving a pair of black leather walking shoes. Both the 1941- and 1943-pattern boots had calves lined with thirty layers of parachute silk to help make them splinter-proof.

In the first two years of the war there is considerable evidence of Bomber Crews' wearing Irvin harness suits. Another option to the 1940 overall and inner lining was the famous Irvin thermally insulated suit made by the Irvin Parachute Company. The fleece-lined jacket and trousers were made from glazed sheepskin and were widely used by bomber crews. Their only disadvantage was that they were sometimes rather bulky for the confined areas of a bomber. Some Irvin suits were wired so that electrically heated gloves and socks could be attached. From 1943 Irvin suits were no longer issued, but they continued to be used in the RAF for many years and are still used today by pilots of vintage aircraft. As well as electrically heated gloves and socks, wired waistcoats were available to bomber crew members sitting in particularly cold parts of the aircraft, such as the 'Tail-end Charlie' in the rear turret. However, electrical supplies, especially to rear turrets, failed so frequently that these men did much better to rely on the thermally insulated Irvin suit or the Taylor buoyant suit. Introduced in July 1942, the Taylor suit was to become a familiar sight in Bomber Command. Tee Emm* says, 'Really warm gunners wear those chic yellow kapok-lined buoyant suits ("You too can have a figure like mine") which pack their own flotation pads, and make Mae West superflous'. These suits were made of a yellow fabric, heavily lined with kapok pads to provide buoyancy.

*Tee Emm–A magazine published by the Air Ministry to give guidance and information to personnel.

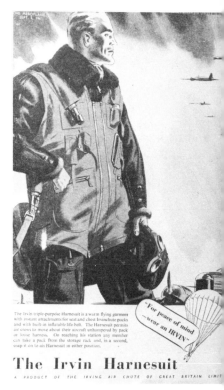

The Irvin triple-purpose Harnesuit is a warm flying garment with instant attachments for seat and chest Irvinchute packs and with built-in inflatable life-belt. The Harnesuit permits air crews to move about their aircraft unhampered by pack or loose harness. On reaching his station any member can take a pack from the storage rack and, in a second, snap it on to his Harnesuit in either position.

The Irvin Harnesuit

A PRODUCT OF THE IRVING AIR CHUTE OF GREAT BRITAIN LIMIT

"For peace of mind — wear an IRVIN"

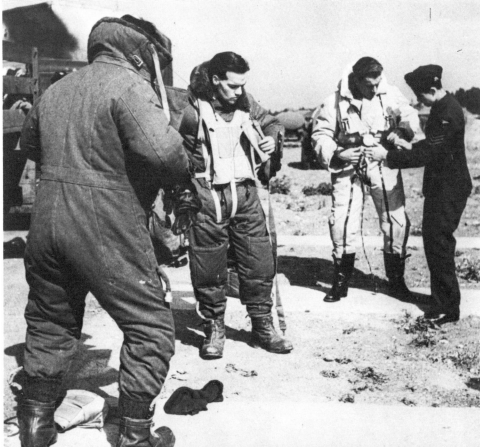

Fortress crew from Polebrook. The two on the left appear to be wearing American or Canadian clothing which is electrically heated. The crewmen on the right is wearing the bulky, yellow Taylor Suit and 1936 Pattern boots.

The Taylor buoyant suit was very warm and provided protection in case of ditching or baling out into the sea – a very real hazard for bomber crews – but was so very bulky that it was unpopular. Electrically heated linings were fitted for mid-upper and rear-gunners. Guy Gibson's rear-gunner, Flight Lieutenant Algernon Trevor-Roper, DFM, used to wear a 'teddy-bear' flying suit in the Lancaster. These were Canadian supplied and worn a lot in Sunderlands. It was not until late in 1944 that hot-air pipes were extended to the rear turret of a Lancaster.

Whitley, Wellington, Lancaster and Halifax bombers had liquid-cooled Merlin engines. This sytem provided heat for the crew, but in spite of this their face, hands, fingers, toes and feet frequently suffered from frostbite. To prevent facial frostbite crews often did not shave for six hours before a flight, in order to leave the protective oils in the skin. Lanolin and other greases were applied, until this was advised against by the Air Ministry in 1944, because the grease could contain water particles, which would increase the chances of frostbite. Carelessness was discouraged while boarding aircraft in full kit in the rain, as

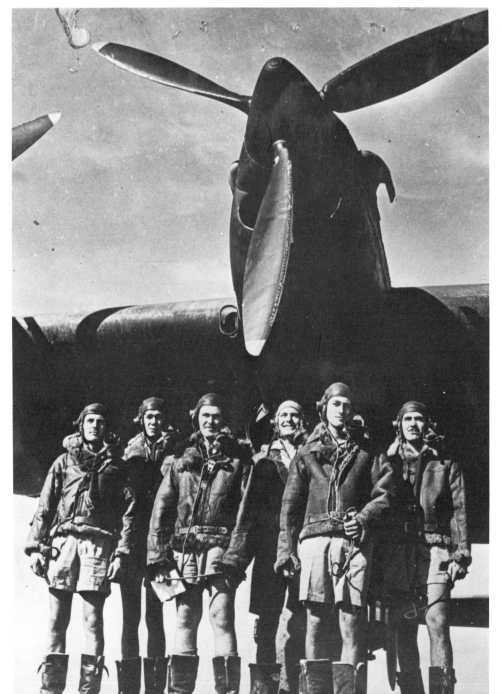

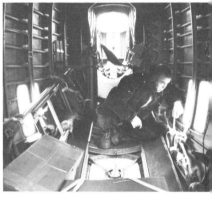

The crew of a Halifax showing the clothing worn by bomber crew in the Middle East campaigns. Only one crewman is wearing the 1936 Pattern boots, the rest have the 1941 Pattern boots without the familiar ankle strap.

A Canadian Teddy Bear Suit worn with the American A-6 boots.

wet clothing was another potential source of frostbite. Aircrew cloakrooms were established to ensure that flying clothing was stored at suitable temperatures for use. The freezing conditions, often $-30°C$, were exacerbated by hypoxia. One Whitley on a leaflet-dropping mission had a defect in the oxygen apparatus which caused a shortage of supply.

> Such was the condition of the navigator and wireless operator at this stage, that every few minutes they were compelled to lie down and rest on the floor of the fuselage. The cockpit heating system was useless. Everyone was frozen and had no means of alleviating their distress. The navigator and Commanding Officer were butting their heads on the floor and navigation table in an endeavour to experience some other form of pain as a relief from the awful feeling of frostbite and lack of oxygen.

There is another story of a Lancaster which in an attack on Berlin lost part of its nose. In normal circumstances the cockpit of an aircraft, which draws its heating from the engines, is quite comfortably warm and the crew 'up-front' are not particularly heavily clothed. However, on this occasion an unbroken stream of icy air surged through the cockpit all the way home. When the plane landed the pilot's hands were frozen to the controls and as a result of this frostbite he lost two fingers.

The 'bends'

Conditions in B-17 Flying Fortresses were even worse as these aircraft flew at very great altitudes, often over 30,000ft, where the cold was more acute and the need for oxygen critical. If a man removed his gloves and touched any metal his flesh would freeze instantly and adhere to it. A distinct shortage of heavy bombers at the beginning of the war led Britain in 1940 to invest in some B-17s from America. These aircraft had a service ceiling, with full load, of 36,700ft, way beyond that of any British bomber. The Stirling could reach only 14,000ft with a full bomb load. The Flying Fortress posed new problems for service flying, problems encountered mainly in record-breaking, high-altitude flights—intense cold, hypoxia and dysbarism (the 'bends'). The bends is a condition which exists in the body when gases, dissolved in the blood and tissues, come out of solution in the form of bubbles. This occurs when the pressure acting on the body decreases, as with altitude. The risk of bends is always present above 30,000ft in unpressurised aircraft. The effects can be crippling if the bubbles lodge in critical parts of the body.

More crew from 90 Squadron showing Type B helmets, Type E masks, MKIIIA goggles, electrically heated suits, Irvin parachute harnesses and American life saving jackets.

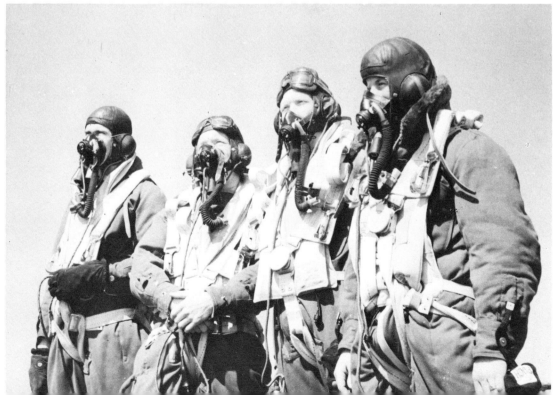

These bubbles of nitrogen which cause the bends, when they have reached the brain, have proved fatal in pressure-chamber 'flights'. The aircrew for Fortresses (No 90 Squadron at Polebrook) were specially selected, under twenty-nine years of age, slightly built and very fit. They were required to sit in the decompression chamber at a simulated altitude of between 32,000 and 35,000 ft for four hours; those susceptible to the bends were rejected.

Fortunately for all Allied operational aircrew a Flying Personnel Research Committee had been formed in 1939 on the advice of Air Marshal Sir Victor Richardson and under the chairmanship of Sir Edward Mellenby. This committee laid out a basic programme of research into the medical problems of service flying, but only eight months after its formation Britain was at war. The RAF Physiological Laboratory, then in a hut at Hendon, moved to Farnborough where Group Captain S. Marshall was joined by Dr B. H. C. Matthews, who headed the research team for the rest of the war. Thankfully the value of aviation medicine was now realised, for a man could not fly or fight well if collapsing through cold or hypoxia.

Doctors flying with aircrews collected information for all manner of improvements necessary to successful missions, and came to appreciate at first hand the desperate strain experienced by flying personnel. Sadly many lost their lives in the course of these duties.

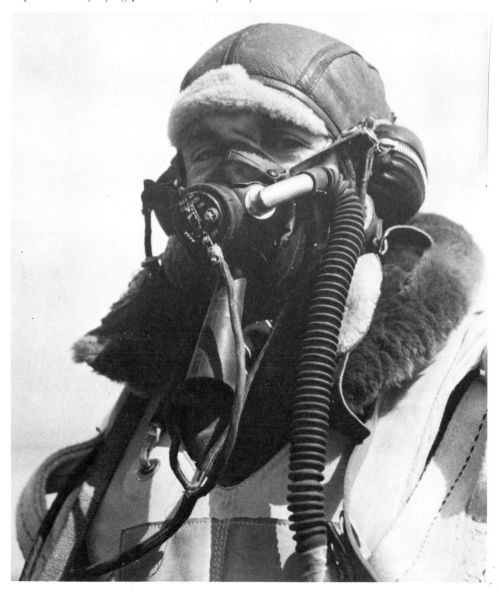

A 90 Squadron crewman poses for the camera. His clothing is a good example of the improvisations made in the early years of the war. The helmet is American but has 22C/66 ear pieces attached at an unusual angle. The oxygen mask is the first of the rubber masks officially issued and has fastenings appropriate to the Type B helmet. We presume that this is the Type E mask having a metal surround to the mask and the aluminium oxygen pipe entering the side of the mask.

No theatre of action was beyond the sphere of the 'lab'. The team immediately began work on efficient and economical oxygen systems. At the beginning of the war the Type D fabric mask and the constant-flow system of oxygen were used but this was an extremely wasteful system as the gas flowed continuously during inhalation and exhalation. Late in 1941 the economiser system was produced whereby gas was released only when the

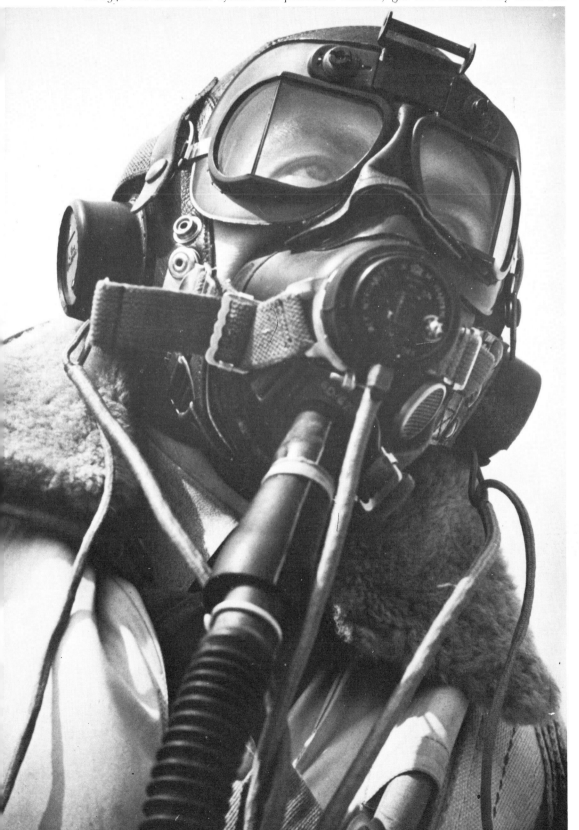

In this view the 90 Squadron crewman is wearing a Type C helmet with external wiring, a Type E* oxygen mask and Mark VII goggles. The oxygen supply enters from the bottom. The positioning straps are suited to the Type C helmet introduced late in 1941. This type of mask harness was elasticated and was used also on the Type G mask.

Note side vent.

man breathed in, and if for any reason the breathing became shallow the pressure would increase enough to open the valve and automatically give a supply.

The very serious effects of oxygen starvation or hypoxia—carefree elation, outbursts of laughter or abuse, violent actions and eventually weakness of limbs, failure of rational thought and unconsciousness were to be found in all phases of operational flying during the war and were the cause of many an accident. Because oxygen canisters meant extra weight, an aircraft frequently did not have an adequate supply for all crew members. In the first year of the war a Hampden aircraft with an endurance of ten hours, carried only enough oxygen for four hours sixteen minutes at or above 15,000 ft. They were using the continuous-flow system and even with extra 750-litre bottles, the supply and flight duration were not in parity. One operation which took place in September 1941 illustrates the disastrous results of hypoxia. Four RAF Fortresses from 90 Squadron took off from Kinloss to bomb the German *Admiral von Scheer* in Oslo Harbour. They headed towards the target at 26,000 ft across the North Sea; one aircraft had been delayed, so only three aircraft were in loose formation. The formation was attacked by Me109s; one Fortress avoided interception and returned safely, a second was shot down, the third aircraft continued. The captain ordered the crew to have their parachutes ready and climbed to 35,000 ft, releasing his bomb load before turning for home. With the distortion of the voice at altitude one of the waist-gunners misunderstood this order, disconnected his oxygen-mask tube from the main supply and plugged it into his emergency portable bottle. Within a few minutes he collapsed. His companion, seeing him collapse, moved to his aid, failing to connect his portable bottle correctly; he, too, passed out in a matter of seconds. For fifteen minutes the two gunners remained unconscious in the rear, until the wireless operator told the pilot they had passed out; the pilot dived the aircraft. At 29,000 ft they were attacked by a German fighter from astern. The ten-second burst of fire hit both gunners; one died of a haemorrhage, the other suffered a wounded hand.

The wireless operator became unconscious when a cannon shell shattered his oxygen pipe. Smoke filled the fuselage, clearing only when the Astro-dome was jettisoned; the fighter, thinking the Fortress on fire, broke off the attack, leaving the stricken aircraft. The ailerons were inoperative and bomb doors would not close. A crew member started to wind the doors up manually but collapsed when his portable oxygen supply gave out. The second pilot connected him to a fresh supply and he soon recovered and continued, while connected to the main supply, to wind the doors up. The economiser did not produce enough oxygen for these exertions and he fainted. The aircraft eventually returned on two engines. It was medically recommended that high-altitude flying be limited to two operations per week as crews tended to become lethargic and irritable after flying at 30,000 ft. A report made by the two doctors with No 90 Squadron recommended that crews should be kept warm and at rest as much as possible, that orders should be repeated twice over the intercom. at altitude, that oxygen-equipment drill should be practised, and that flights in excess of 35,000 ft should be made only in aircraft fitted with pressurised cabins.

Experimental work continued at Farnborough, Dr Gilson and Miss M. Worthington making significant contributions to the development of oxygen systems. As a result of the experience gained on the Fortresses, it was evident that more work was needed on masks, and these two members of the establishment involved themselves with the problems. Collecting information from flights in Harrows, Wellingtons and, later, Lancasters, as well as making experiments in the decompression chamber, they ascertained the rate of oxygen consumption necessary to perform aircrew duties in flight. The extremely low temperatures at high altitude led to the exposure of another problem; the masks used with the economiser proved to freezing up. As a result of extensive tests in the altitude chamber at Farnborough Dr Gilson produced redesigned mask, the Type E*, which not only avoided icing in the valves but also decreased the mask's size to improve vision. There then followed the Type F and Type G masks. The Type G mask was so designated in April 1941 although production did not commence until 1942. Supplies were limited until 1943 when in April of that year 13,000 were produced. With anti-dematitic internal finish the masks were well liked. During 1943 work was commenced on the Type H mask.

Reconnaissance flying

Mention should be made here of the high-altitude, photo-reconnaissance squadrons that flew over enemy-occupied territory to glean information for Bomber Command. These flights posed all the classic problems of high-altitude flying. During the 1939–40 'phoney war' period, efforts were being made to build up the number of photo-reconnaissance squadrons with Mk1 Spitfires, stripped of all unnecessary equipment to increase the aircraft's range and altitude capabilities. The successful increase demanded an oxygen system of enlarged capacity. The Type D fabric masks of that period gave a poor seal around the face, and the constant-flow oxygen system was extremely wasteful. Late in 1941 the RAF team produced the economiser system, and the Type F rubber mask was developed which reduced all leaks around the face. This system effectively doubled the range of the early reconnaissance aircraft.

In 1942 Ju86P aircraft were operating over the Nile Delta, and interceptions were attempted in modified Mk V Spitfires at altitudes in excess of 40,000 ft; no special pressure clothing was worn but remarkably several attempts at interception were successful. The Ju86s posed a serious threat when they began to operate over Britain as they could photograph at will the preparations for D-Day. The Mk VI Spitfire, of which 100 were built, had a pressurised cockpit, so that the cabin altitude at 40,000 ft was the equivalent of only 28,000 ft. Two squadrons of Spitfire Mk IX were modified to enable them to fly at high altitudes, but they were not pressurised, and there remained the probability of a high incidence of bends and anoxia. Some interceptions were successful and the Ju86 problem ceased; but pilots still had to carry out high-altitude photo-reconnaissance for Bomber Command.

Pressurised Spitfires were used for photo-reconnaissance as well as for interception, beginning with the production of sixteen unarmed Mk X Spitfires. Pilots did not like them, as the power required to pressurise the cabin reduced the engine power. The canopies also fogged up, a hazard the Germans avoided in the Ju86 by having double hermetically sealed panes with water-absorbent calcium chloride pellets inserted. The Mk XVI Mosquito, which flew in 1943, suffered from the same disadvantages. The Mk XIX Spitfire, with a 2,050-hp Griffon engine, and the Mosquito 34 were both types which had much greater power and satisfied the photo-reconnaissance requirements well. The Germans pressurised some Me109Gs and were working on the FwTa152H when the war came to an end. In the absence of pressure cabins or full-pressure suits, the only protection against the bends was the careful selection of pilots.

Air pressure problems

At heights above 37,000 ft the decrease in barometric pressure is such that even with 100 per cent oxygen, the pressure in the lungs is too low to force the gas into solution in the blood. In 1942 Professor H. C. Bazett, then working in Canada, was asked to join the Flying Personnel Research Committee. Professor Bazett had become an expert in the problems of respiration at great altitudes; he conceived the idea of 'pressure-breathing', the principle being that by breathing out of the oxygen mask against a predetermined positive pressure, the oxygen saturation into the blood must increase. To make breathing less laborious he applied a counter-pressure to the chest by means of a waistcoat, which was pressurised by the oxygen supply into the garment and at the same time acted as a reservoir of supply to the oxygen mask. Development work went on in the laboratories and chambers at Farnborough. It became certain that the equipment would enable photo-reconnaissance pilots to fly at 44,000 ft for thirty minutes, which would give them a considerable advantage over the German defences. Two squadrons using this equipment successfully brought back photographs of V1 and V2 sites.

The system devised by Professor Bazett provided a pressure of $\frac{1}{4}$ lb per sq. in. in the mask and lungs, which was satisfactory up to 44,000 ft; higher altitudes indicated the need to increase the pressure to $\frac{1}{2}$ lb per sq. in. The potential need for increased pressures presented physiological problems. In the decompression chamber at Farnborough, Professor Bazett experimented on himself using his own pressure-breathing waistcoat and an original water-filled anti-'G' suit–the Franks flying suit. Thus equipped he managed to stay at 50,000 ft for twenty minutes without incident.

Vision research

It was in Bomber and Coastal Commands that the problems of vision fatigue, night vision, searchlight dazzle and airsickness were most apparent. After the Battle of Britain the German bomber force operated at night, resulting in a necessary increase in our own night-fighter force. At the same time our own bomber force was enlarged and was engaged in offensives further into occupied territory. A situation developed where both the attacker and defender had to have the best in vision for his nocturnal activities.

It was found that dark goggles worn half an hour before a flight meant a great improvement in visual acuity at night. However, these dark goggles made life in the crew room rather tedious so, after experiment, goggles with ruby-red lenses were found effective for improving night vision without restricting the wearers' normal domestic activities. Instruments and cockpit lighting were devised to help keep 'night vision' to a maximum. Oxygen, or rather the lack of oxygen, affected sight more by night than by day. The surprisingly low altitude of 4,000 ft was critical, so crews used oxygen from the ground up to their operating altitudes. It was found that a rear-gunner using oxygen in this way had his night vision improved by as much as forty per cent.

Air Commodore Livingstone, a foremost authority in the field of vision research, spent much of his time working on the problems of pilot vision and orientation. His inventiveness led him to develop a device to test acceptable standards of aircrew vision, and a means of determining those pilots who had a special aptitude for night work. He also spent time on the development of special goggles to reduce glare from searchlights. In 1940 it was suggested that tinted, shatter-proof goggles of the type used in the Middle and Far East be introduced for bomber crews. In 1941 air-gunners were issued with Mk-IVB and VA goggles with tinted visors. Only 2,000 Mk-VA goggles were produced as the Supply Branch argued that a general air-crew goggle, Mk VI, be produced. Modified ski-ing goggles were tried out by crews of 3 Group, but there were problems with supply. In October 1941 Dr Livingstone tried developing spectacles to relieve eyestrain, particularly for pilots. Pilot Officer Lloyd of No 83 Squadron wore these spectacles on several missions and reported that the frames impeded vision, and offered no advantages over issued goggles. Full tests were curtailed when Pilot Officer Lloyd failed to return from a raid.

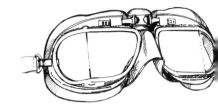

MKVIII goggles were introduced in 19.. and were worn until the 1960's by certa.. aircrew.

Fire

Bomber crews, like their fighter colleagues, feared the hazard of fire more than the ever-present problems of cold, fatigue, oxygen starvation and the difficulty of night vision. In September 1940, No 83 Squadron was detailed to raid the docks at Antwerp, which was crammed with barges for 'Operation Sealion'. As a Hampden roared over the docks a shell crashed into the aircraft. The rear-gunner's cockpit became a roaring inferno and the rear-gunner took to his parachute, landing safely. The fire swept forward, fed by rushing air, and reached the wireless operator's compartment occupied by Sergeant Hannah. The captain asked for a damage report and advised the crew to stand by to abandon the aircraft. Hannah, surrounded by flames, grabbed the first thing to hand, the radio log book. He attempted to beat out the flames, which only got worse. The ammunition in the gunner's cockpit exploded sending bullets around the aircraft, and fuel from fractured pipes gushed into the fuselage. Hannah's only chance was to get an extinguisher in the forward compartment, behind the aluminium door which had jammed. In despair he flung himself on the door and broke it down, bouncing off he fell into the flames behind him. Wriggling free he grabbed one of the extinguishers which he sprayed on to the fire.

Suffocating in the fumes – his oxygen pipe was disconnected and a portable bottle was out of the question in view of the speed at which everything was happening – he continued to fight the fire. It now broke out in the bomb bay, melting the floor as Hannah reached for the other extinguisher, and burning the soles off his flying boots. With his head swimming he tore off his oxygen mask, with the result that his face was burnt by the fierce wall of fire. With his gloves burnt off he continued until the extinguisher was exhausted and the fire abated, beating out what flames remained with his hands and feet.

After this he opened the escape hatch above his head and threw out burning fragments. Terribly burnt, he reported to the captain that the fire was out. However, their troubles were not over, as the aircraft was badly crippled and the navigator had also baled out. Together they somehow got the aircraft back to base. Following a series of operations Sergeant Hannah recovered and was awarded the VC for his tremendous bravery.

One reassurance for a bomber pilot was that he had armour plating to protect him, a luxury fighter pilots did not receive until later in the war. A Lancaster pilot had an armoured seat-back and piece of bullet-proof glass behind his head. However, the remaining crew members were not so lucky; and to try to lessen the number of ghastly injuries caused by cannon shell and shrapnel, trials were carried out by No 44 Squadron in December 1943, using American flak-suits, helmets and Army body-armour, which was general issue to ground troops. A report made by the squadron and received in March 1944 indicated that crews disliked wearing these garments and that the helmet was too heavy and cumbersome for wear when moving around an aircraft in total darkness. These innovations were not adopted.

Crew of a Boston aircraft wearing a Trans-atlantic mixture of clothing. Three are wearing RAF battle dress and 1943 black escape boots with American flak suits and special M-4 flak helmets which fit over the normal Type C helmet.

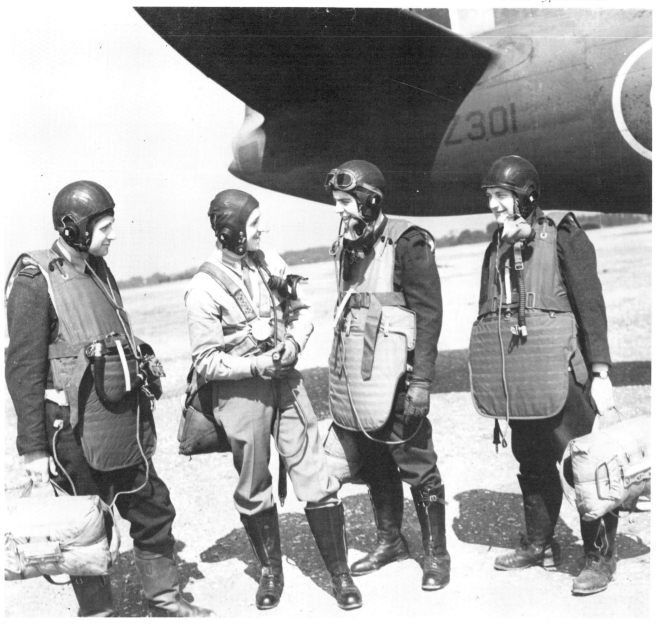

Survival kit

Bomber crews had the fearful awareness that they were most of the time over enemy-occupied territory, a stimulus not shared by men of Coastal Command who had the tedious job of touring the endless no-man's-land of ocean. Crews of Coastal Command aircraft could expect flights lasting from two hours in a Tiger Moth in 1939 up to nineteen hours in a Liberator in 1944. They were continuously searching the watery wastes for lost crews of aircraft and sunken ships, for enemy convoys and battleships; they patrolled our own convoys and were always on the look-out for the periscope wake of an unwary submarine.

Aircrews of Coastal Command were issued with standard RAF flying clothing, although eccentricities crept in. Because of the reliance on visual contacts and the corresponding low altitudes flown, the problem of cold was much reduced. Flying for many hours at a time was no great problem as bunk beds were provided so that off-duty crew could rest, and they were able to cook meals on a small stove. Oxygen equipment was supplied but rarely used; masks were primarily worn for communication. One of the main problems for Coastal Command crew was the fierce glare reflected off the sea. In 1943 special Polaroid spectacles were introduced, which were very effective.

The crew of a Coastal Command Hudson board their aircraft, 1941. They are al wearing Irvin harness suits and have Type L helmets and Type D masks.

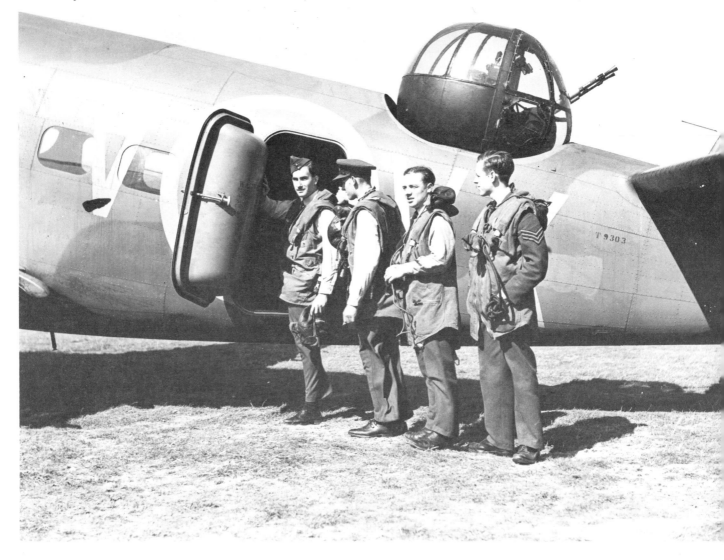

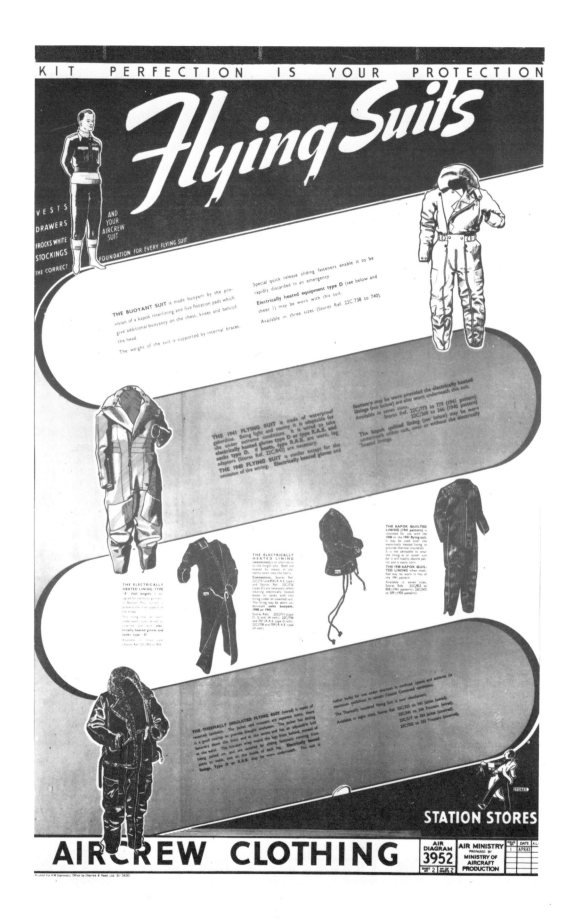

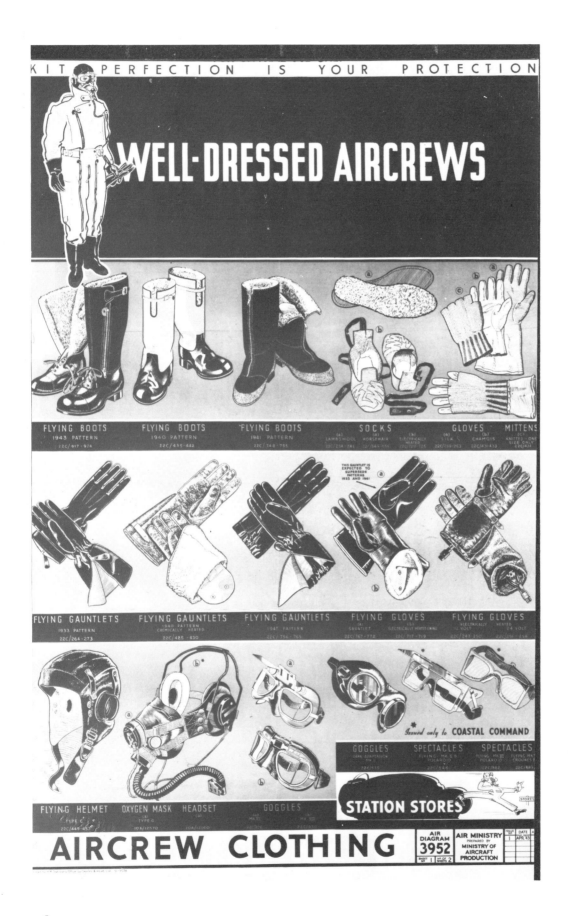

Because of the long distances flown over the sea at low altitudes, great reliance was placed on the 'Mae West', or life-jacket, named after the famous film star. Materials like cork and kapok had been used in flotation jackets, in fact the Germans still issued kapok life-jackets to their bomber crews. These jackets were bulky because obviously the more cork or kapok used the greater the flotation achieved. They were, therefore, unacceptable in the small working spaces of most aircraft. So a flat life-jacket with inflatable rubber bladders was introduced, the Mae West. These bladders were inflated in an emergency by the wearer, but as from about 1941 a small bottle of compressed CO_2 was provided for this purpose. Squadron Leader E. A. Pask did much work on the development of this life-jacket so that it not only kept a man from sinking but also, if he were unconscious, would keep his nose and mouth clear of the water.

Air warfare over the sea provided many problems of survival, for even if one managed to bale out or ditch into the sea without injury one's chances of surviving for long in the icy waters of the North Atlantic were slim, and hypothermia, or critical loss of body heat, soon set in. One project assigned to Squadron Leader Pask was the protection of pilots assigned to Catapult-Aircraft Merchantmen ships, the duty of these pilots being to provide fighter protection to convoys in the North Atlantic. Hurricanes catapulted from CAM ships would intercept Focke-Wolf Condors flying from Norway, if possible shoot them down, then ditch in the sea. The Air Ministry considered that it was worth losing one fighter in order to save merchant ships which were defenceless against the bombing raids of the Condors.

In the North Atlantic in winter, temperatures were so low that a man would die of exposure in a few minutes. Some form of suit had to be designed which would protect the wearer until he could be picked up. The first thoughts were concentrated on what type of material could be used. It was essential that it should 'breathe', but become waterproof when immersed in water. Horse leather offered a suitable solution, but after successful tests it was found to be impossible to produce these suits in quantity. Material used for making portable water tanks was obtained which had the same properties as horse leather, but was readily available. The design of rubber seals round the neck, hands and feet proved difficult, but suits were eventually available for test. Dr Pask, wearing the suit with attached rubber boots, proved its worth on a test in the sea off the Shetland Isles. The trial had to be terminated because the crew of the launch could not tolerate the cold. The suit was proved, but long-range air cover was now available for convoys, and the need for CAM fighters ceased. Both the Navy and Bomber Command carried out trials with this suit, the former adopting it and proceeding with its further development.

American intervention

Early in the morning of 7 December 1941 the Japanese took an unforeseen step. With a large force of bomber, torpedo and fighter aircraft, they attacked the American Pacific Fleet at anchor in Pearl Harbour. The repercussions of this act were to be played out in all theatres of the war. America declared war on Japan and at the same time resolved to pursue greater activity in the European theatre.

The American concept of strategic bombing was essentially different from that of the RAF. They aimed to specialise in long-range daylight raids, using altitude to minimise the danger of anti-aircraft fire and fighter interception. A superb bomb sight allowed them, in good visibility, to accurately bomb targets from average altitudes of between 27,000 and 30,000 ft. The aeroplane that initially made this possible was the Boeing B17 Flying Fortress, so called because of the great number of ·5 machine-guns carried for defence. B17Cs, known as the Fortress I in the RAF, were flown by the RAF at altitudes of up to 39,000 ft on a number of daylight raids. The losses sustained caused the Boeing Company to modify the design and produce the B17E. These aircraft were in US service at the time of Pearl Harbour, together with the Convair B24 Liberator.

Based in the eastern parts of England, the US 8th Air Force began in 1942 to stage offensive raids in daylight against Germany, using close defensive formations and high-altitude bombing techniques. Losses were small in the initial raids, mainly because the bombers did not operate beyond the range of the escorting Spitfires supplied by the RAF.

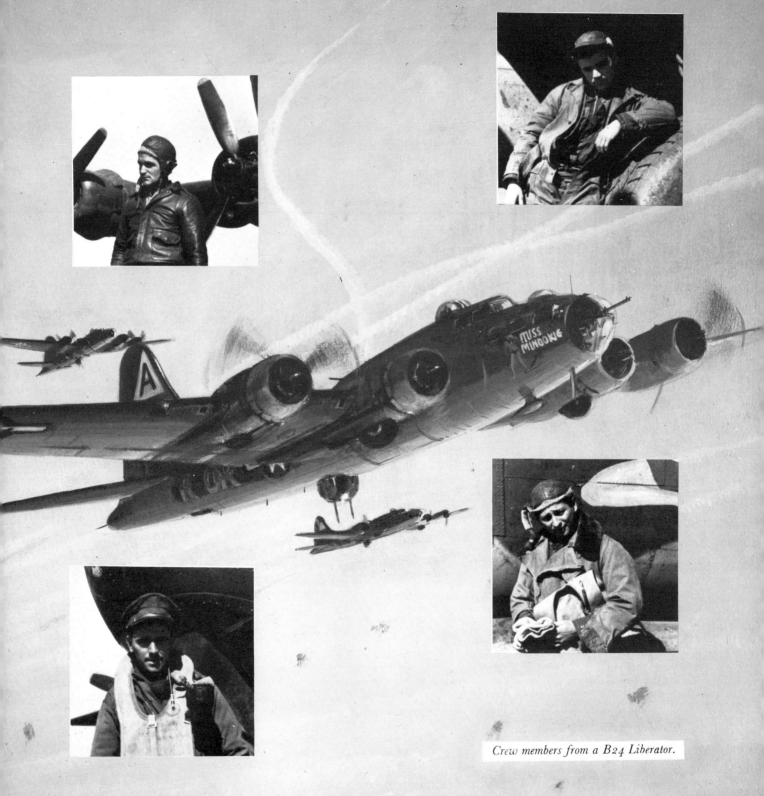

Crew members from a B24 Liberator.

After the Casablanca Conference of January 1943 a joint daylight- and night-bombing policy was evolved between the 8th Air Force and Bomber Command which led to a rapid increase in aircraft and crews and the build-up of massive daylight offensive plans. In 1943 large formations of B24s and B17s were sent on long-range missions over Germany. Losses rose considerably as soon as the bombers left the protection of the Spitfires and the American P38 and P47 fighters, now also based in England. The *Luftwaffe*, now on the alert, increased their fighter defences to cope with these raids, using fighters equipped with cannons, rockets, machine-guns and mortars. The RAF's advantage in the Battle of Britain was now the *Luftwaffe*'s, who were fighting on their own soil, no longer hampered by operating range. Fighters could attack in-bound bombers, land, re-fuel, and attack the same bomber as it returned.

Naval aviators, students from the Corpus Christi Naval Air Station. From L. to R. the Naval green uniform, the lightweight jacket, the light coverall for warm weather, the medium jacket, the heavy jacket and finally a fur-lined Shearling suit for high altitude flying.

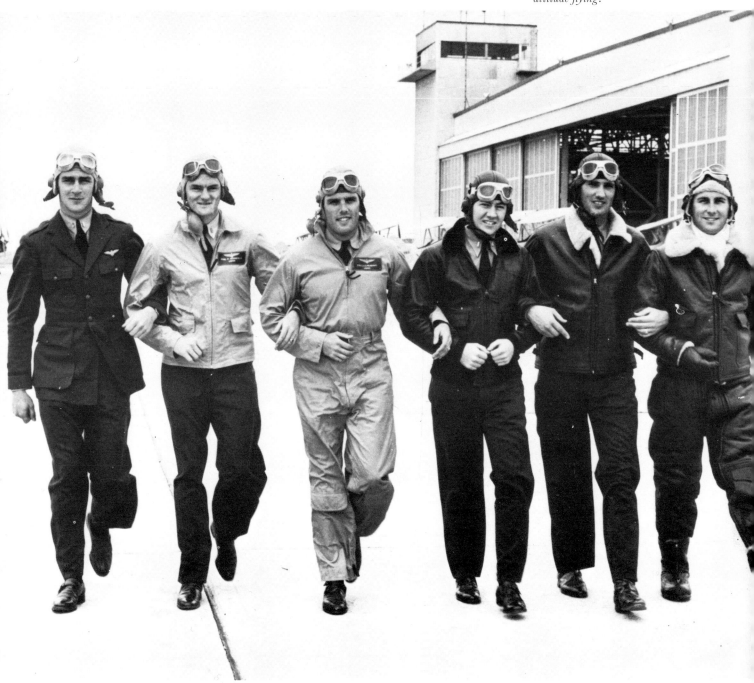

The *Luftwaffe* was in a superior position, but this situation was not to last. P47 fighters, equipped with drop-tanks, were able to keep with the bombers for much greater distances over occupied territories. These fighters were joined by the P51 Mustang, which was probably the most successful fighter aircraft of the war. With drop-tanks its range was excellent, and with the Merlin engine it out-performed all contemporary fighters. With a full escort system to back up the increasing stream of B24 and B17 bomber aircraft the 8th Air Force proceeded to hammer the *Third Reich* daily for the next two years. America also took a hand in affairs in the Western Desert. The 9th Air Force, first operating B24s from Western Desert strips, then using Mitchell and Marauder medium bombers as well, fought their way through Italy to join the 8th Air Force.

To oversee the health of the thousands of aircrewmen engaged by the American air services across the world was a considerable problem. Before the war American flight surgeons had been through a flying training programme, but in war time, with an accelerated training scheme carried out at the School of Aviation Medicine at Randolph Field, Texas, only ten hours' dual flying was given in training aircraft. The field work carried out by these trained men was backed up by the Aero Medical Laboratory at Wright Field, Ohio, the Army Air Force School of Aviation Medicine and the Navy School of Aviation Medicine. To supplement the work of these establishments medical schools and medical centres also contributed to research programmes.

Oxygen supply

One of the major problems to be solved was the adequate supply of oxygen to crews who were bombing by day at altitudes of between 25,000 and 30,000ft. There were many fatal accidents in 1942 as a result of faulty or inadequate equipment. Initially in B17E aircraft, crews wore the A8 mask, linked to an A8A constant-flow regulator. This thin, moulded rubber mask had been developed at the Mayo Clinic in 1938 by Boothby, Lovelace and Bulbulian. The mask had sponge-rubber-filled parts which allowed exhalation to the atmosphere; a re-breather bag was also involved. With a small quantity of oxygen filling the bag at low altitudes, the bag would be exhausted before the lungs filled so the rubber parts in the mask allowed air to enter to complete inspiration. This was a basic-dilution system. When operating under stress and at altitude, the regulator setting had to be changed. This could cause problems if a crew man did not hear the captain's warning to change regulator settings. Another hazard with the A8 mask was that moisture exhaled through the parts in the mask, would freeze at high altitudes. Because of this the 8th Air Force ordered that a spare mask be issued for each member of a crew, and missions would not be flown higher than 25,000ft. In 1940 the RAF took possession of many German Auer demand regulators. Captain Otis Benson Jr, MC obtained some examples which were worked on by the Aero Medical Laboratory at Wright Field in 1941. These led to the American A12 diluter demand regulator which was issued in 1944. It provided the right air/oxygen mixture automatically to altitudes exceeding 34,000ft. The A12 regulator had low-pressure, shatter-proof cylinders and was issued with the A9 and A10 masks which did not freeze up readily. These masks were copied by the Germans. The A14 mask was issued to American fighter pilots, whose cockpit temperatures were higher than those in bomber aircraft, thus eliminating their tendency to freeze. Temperatures at 20,000ft can be as low as $-76°$F.

American clothing

American bombers carried a crew of ten as opposed to the seven crew members in RAF heavy bombers. They had a considerable problem in keeping warm, for the air-cooled engines meant that petrol-fuelled stoves had to be installed in their aircraft to offer some cheer. Faulty equipment and lack of experience led to chronic cases of frostbite. Bare flesh froze instantly when in contact with metal surfaces at 67° of frost. Silk or cotton gloves prevented moisture from the skin contacting the cold metal. Gunners removing gloves to clear jammed guns or change oxygen masks were the most frequent sufferers.

Waist-gunners had no protection for their faces until plexiglass windows, which allowed the guns freedom of movement, were introduced to the 8th Air Force in 1944. Both turret-gunners, left in their positions for up to eight hours, had to urinate in their clothing, suffering terrible frostbite of the thighs and buttocks. It was not until 1940 that development started on electrically heated suits. The General Electric and US Rubber Companies manufactured sixteen suits which were tested in unheated P40 aircraft at high altitude. The General Electric suits proved the more successful and were standardised as the Type E1 for twelve volts and F1 for twenty-four volts. Despite problems of injury from breakages of wire in these suits, 80,000 were ordered. The Engineering Section at Wright Field stated that in June 1941 no aircraft had sockets or electrical supplies for the suits. However, sockets would be provided for tail- and turret-gunners in B17, B24, B25 and B26 aircraft. By July 1941 100 twenty-four volt F1 suits were procured for B17s and 12,000 twelve-volt suits were also ordered; eventually 80,000 suits were available, but on account of failures few were available to crews.

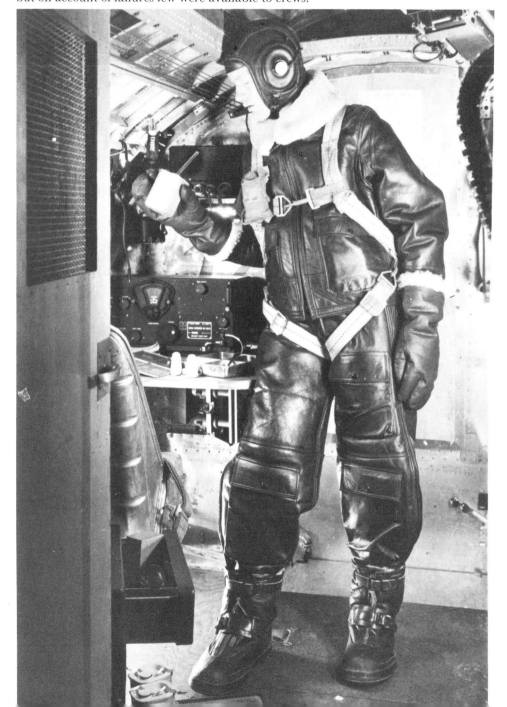

USAAF radio operator in Shearling flying clothing. His outfit includes a Type AN-H-16 helmet, AN-J-4 jacket, AN-T-35 trousers, and A-6 boots with straps.

These electrically heated under-suits were unreliable because of constant breakages in the heating elements. Burns were common and yet at the same time the back, hands and feet would often freeze. Suits were wired in series, so if one element failed the entire suit stopped working. Modifications were clearly necessary. Colonel A. P. Gagge of the Aero Medical Laboratory made a report on the operations of the 8th Air Force. He found that during the winter of 1943–4, the number of American Air Force bombers actually carrying out bomber raids was determined more by the amount of adequate clothing available than by any other cause. Of all casualties returning from missions with the 8th Air Force fifty per cent were suffering from frostbite. The first suit capable of giving comfortable warmth in temperatures as low as −60°F was the F3, a two-piece cotton-and-rayon twill suit introduced in March 1944. The F3 suit had thirteen parallel circuits, two in the jacket, three in the trousers and two in the accompanying shoes and gloves. This allowed the partial operation of the suit if one or more elements were damaged. Development continued with the F3A suit using the British-type, mesh-gauze heating elements, and until the end of World War II the F3 remained standard.

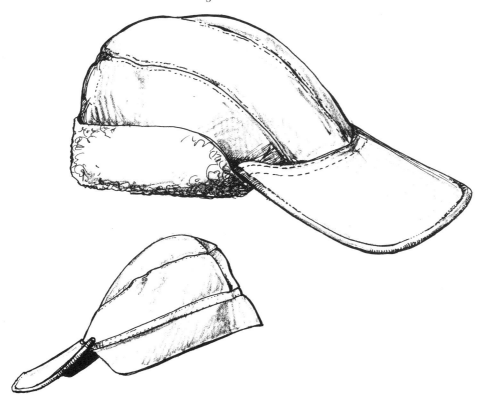

The USAAF Type B-2 helmet. Made fro[m] Shearling material with a stiffened chrom[e] leather peak, it was used a lot by crews [of] bomber and transport aircraft. Headphon[es] were fitted on top of the helmet.

While work was being carried out on the development of an efficient electrically heated suit American airmen wore what was known as the Shearling suit, the equivalent of the RAF Irvin suit. These suits had been developed from the Quartermaster Corps ski- and mountaineering-troop clothing. They were widely used for three years from the winter of 1940. The jacket was designated B6 and the trousers A5. They were made of sheepskin with a pile three-quarters of an inch thick, and seventy-five sq ft of sheepskin was required for each suit. The US Army Air Force required 12,000,000 sq ft of pelts in 1943 alone. Heavy wool vests lined with Shearling were also available.

Shearling suits were by no means ideal for bomber crewmen. They were extremely bulky and cumbersome, making it difficult to move around the aircraft. Their bulky nature also made speedy first aid difficult. Zippers had been incorporated in the suits, but even these posed problems. In spring 1943 slide fasteners were scarce since brass, the best material, was in short supply. As a result zinc and other alloys were tried, but experience showed that hundreds of suits were rendered useless by corrosion of these substitute metals.

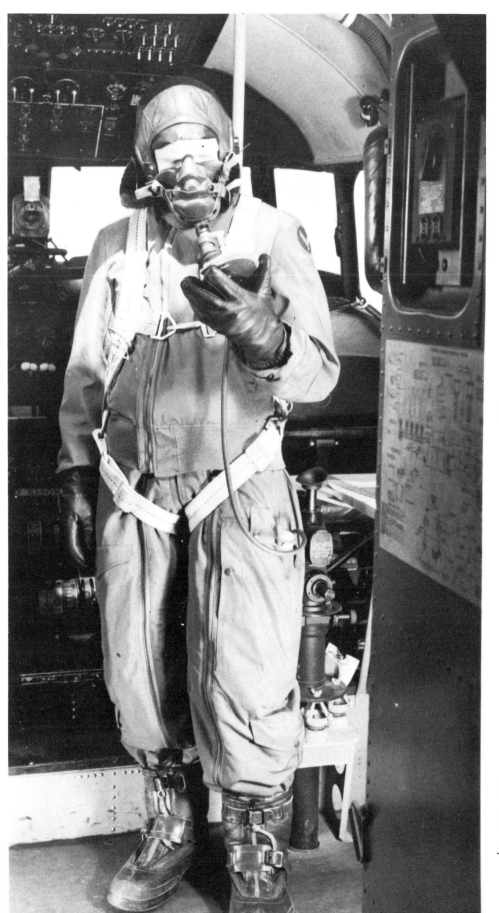

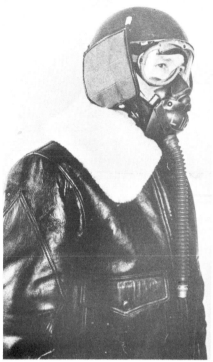

Integration of oxygen mask, goggles and helmet with armoured helmet, 1943. The mask is Type A-14.

USAAF navigator in intermediate flying clothing. His outfit includes Type A-11 helmet, B-15 jacket, A-11 trousers, A-6 boots and A-11 gloves and an A-19 demand mask.

He holds in his left hand the supply tube from an H-1 bailout bottle of oxygen.

In spite of the fact that a lot of money would be lost, it was decided that a change be made from the unsatisfactory Shearling suit to wool and alpaca pile. A combination of A11 trousers with B15 jacket was introduced. At the same time 50,000 quilted down suits (A8 trousers and B9 jacket) were issued. As from March 1944 the B13 flight-jacket, developed at the request of General H. Arnold from the design of the RAF battledress jacket and the Canadian 'Aircrew Suit', was available. Other standard clothing included the B5 Shearling helmet, the A7 summer helmet made of horsehide and lined with chamois, and the unlined gabardine A9 helmet. Many American crews based in England had used the Type C helmet. In 1943 all helmets were replaced by the A11.

A significant innovation in the field of flying clothing was the American 'flak suit'. Armour plating fitted to aircraft was insufficient to shield all crewmen. The more exposed occupants could be torn apart by cannon shells. Flak splinters could maim or kill. In October 1942 Brigadier General M. C. Grow, MC, after discovering that seventy per cent of combat wounds were the result of low-velocity fragments, devised, with the aid of the Wilkinson Sword Company, a vest made of one-mm manganese steel plates which would stop a ·45 bullet at close range. By March 1943 twelve B17 crews were issued with these vests which, in spite of the fact that each of them weighed twenty lb, proved entirely successful. Quantity production was carried out in the USA and by 1944 13,500 flak suits were in use with the 8th Air Force.

Flak suits were not personal issue and were delivered to the aircraft before flight and collected again later for inspection. Aircrew were urged to use the equipment approaching the target area. In emergency a rip cord could be pulled to release the entire suit of body armour.

The flak helmets were personal issue but also had to be returned to the supply room after each flight.

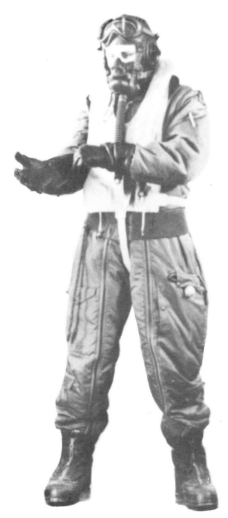

Intermediate Suit with B-8 goggles, A-1 helmet, A-14 mask and standard American life jacket, 1945.

The bailout bottle in the left pocket is an H-1. The pilot should grip the pipe stem between his teeth before leaving the aircraft.

With the later H-2 type it was only necessary to turn the bottle on and release the main oxygen supply hose. The end of this hose should be covered by the left hand until the parachute opens.

These units were considered essential for operations above 30,000 feet.

To complement the suit, an infantry M1 helmet was stretched to accommodate headphones. These helmets were the invention of Colonel Otis C. Benson, Flight-Surgeon with the 12th Bomber Command, later to become the 15th Air Force. An improved version was designed by General Grow. Made from manganese steel and labelled the M4, it was mass produced and issued to the 8th Air Force. By these means casualty figures were successfully reduced.

America again led the way in the introduction of the anti-'G' suit to service. The US Navy developed an anti-'G' suit, referred to as the eighteen-lb Navy suit, which was tested intensively on a centrifuge by the Aero Medical Laboratory at Wright Field. After successful tests the Army Air Force adopted the G3 suit. The suit was basically a pair of pants weighing two lb, containing air bladders; these automatically inflated with compressed air when 'G' force was registered on a specially designed inlet valve. The pressure was automatically released when these 'G' forces ceased. This suit had three compartments, run off the instrument pump, with the same pressure in each compartment. It was stated in 1945, that pilots wearing these suits did not experience blackouts, and that the extra margin of clear-headedness achieved with the suit made a considerable difference to the outcome of aerial combat. Several thousand G3 suits were issued in 1944. This development led to the rescinding of the British decision of 1943, and development of anti-'G' suits on American lines began in 1944.

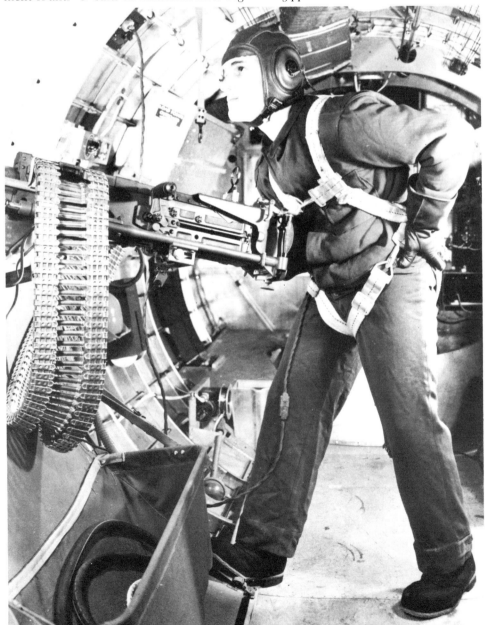

USAAF B-17 waist gunner wearing an F-2 electrically heated flying suit and boots. His helmet is a Type AN-H-16.

Flying fatigue, airsickness and mental breakdowns resulting from the accumulated effects of fear and exhaustion affected very many men flying operationally. This was especially so in the Pacific where long, boring flights had to be made by the Air Force and Navy alike to reach Japanese-held islands and contact enemy aircraft. Many of the aircraft were single-engined machines and offered little chance of movement for the pilot in flights that might be as long as seven hours. Hypoxia and cold were not in these instances such a problem as many flights relied on contact being made with the enemy at low altitude; but with concentration flagging after long hours, little height often remained in which to regain control of aircraft when disorientation set in. Loneliness, helplessness and futility gnawed at the crews of single-plane operations, contributing to the collapse of the airman's mental state. Even with B24s, carrying a crew of ten men on offensive missions, this feeling led to insurmountable anxieties in certain cases.

When the Japanese attacked Pearl Harbour, they had already taken a vast territory of sea and many small islands in the Pacific. The Army Air Force was naturally involved in this conflict, but the major retaliatory action was taken by the US Navy. Their job was to fly fighters and torpedo-aircraft from aircraft-carriers and reduce the Japanese defences on small islands to rubble, seek out and if possible destroy Japanese naval vessels, and generally spearhead American advances across the Pacific towards Tokyo. Although the early encounters with Japanese aircraft proved damaging to the US Navy, it was not long before the initial superiority enjoyed by the Japanese was lost. In the Pacific theatre of war American aircrews wore a lightweight, summer flying suit made from a cotton gabardine.

The Japanese did not install armour-plating in their aircraft; as a result the range and manoeuvrability of the machine were not impaired but the vulnerability was. No self-sealing fuel tanks were supplied, and consequently many Japanese pilots were burned to death or killed by a bullet which would otherwise have been deflected by armour-plate. Japanese aircrews wore a one-piece flying overall with a zip-up front and a belt. They wore leather knee-length flying boots in brown or black and a flying helmet in black, dark brown or light brown. Fur-lined helmets were widely used and fur collars were available for their overalls.

The American Navy operated Grumman F4F Wildcat fighters in 1942, superseded by Grumman Hellcats. These aircraft, along with the Chance-Vought Corsair fighters, were also used in the Pacific conflict by the Australian and New Zealand Air Forces and the Fleet Air Arm. These fighters harried Japanese troops and shipping, and escorted carrier-based bombers and torpedo-aircraft such as the Grumman Avenger and Dauntless. The Japanese retaliated with the Mitsubishi A6M-2 Zero fighter which was a superb aeroplane, if lacking adequate defence. It out-turned and out-climbed the P40 and Wildcat fighters with ease. For their attacks on strategic targets the Japanese had developed a twin-engined bomber with a range of 2,500 miles, the Mitsubishi G4M-1 (Betty), and operated carrier-based torpedo-bombers.

On islands in the Coral Sea the Americans were able to construct airstrips, a facility which gave them the advantage over the Japanese, who relied on flying-boats and sea-planes. The manufacturing might of America began to tell; the Japanese tenaciously held on to almost untenable positions but slowly the borders of their newly acquired empire rolled back towards defeat. In desperation obsolete aircraft were flown by partially trained pilots on suicide missions. The aircraft were deliberately crashed on American ships; it was only a matter of time before the end came for Japan.

The aircraft which delivered the final blow in South-East Asia was the Boeing B29 Superfortress. The B17 and B24 aircraft were not really suitable for action in the Pacific with the vast distances involved, and it was during the early summer of 1944 that their replacement arrived. The design began in 1940 when the Air Force asked for a very heavy bomber, which would carry 2,000 lb of bombs 5,333 miles at 400 mph. The B29 was produced. With a wing span of 141 ft and weighing sixty-two tons, it dwarfed the standard heavy bombers. Like its contemporaries it had a crew of ten men, but they were housed in compartments forward and aft which were pressurised to a differential of 6·55 psi and were connected by a tunnel. The gunners had observation bubbles in the fuselage from which to control their computer gun-sights.

In practice the B29 was an unknown quantity. The Army Air Force had no previous experience with pressurised aircraft. The pressurised system could simulate an altitude of 8,000 ft at 30,000 ft, a relatively high pressure-differential. However, pressure-chamber tests showed that no body damage was sustained by men subjected to 'explosive' decompression, simulating an altitude increase from 8,000 to 30,000 ft in 0·7 seconds, as long as oxygen was being used. This rate of decompression equated to a hole being made in the aircraft's fuselage twelve feet in diameter. In operational service the only instances of decompression involved the fuselage sighting-blisters which were only thirty inches in diameter. As crews were well briefed about wearing oxygen masks, the only man to be seriously injured was Sergeant James Krantz, a gunner aboard the 'American Main', who was blown out of the sighting-blister. Because he was wearing a restraining harness he was eventually pulled back into the aeroplane by crew members.

A Ventura crew from the Royal New Zealand Air Force, wearing clothing typical of the S.E. Asia campaign.

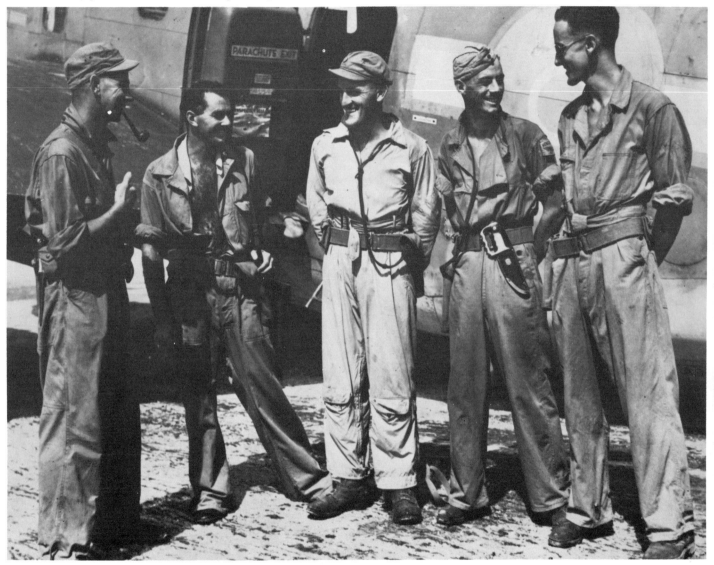

The Germans finally capitulated on 7 May 1945, but the war in the Pacific continued. Resources in Europe started to be diverted to South East Asia. Fortunately they would would not be needed. On 6 August 1945, a lone B29, the *Enola Gay*, flying at 31,600 ft dropped the first atomic bomb on Hiroshima, unopposed, in daylight. Three days later another B29, *Bock's Car*, dropped a second atom bomb on the city of Nagasaki. The release of these terrible weapons forced a speedy Japanese surrender and ended the hideous global conflict of World War II.

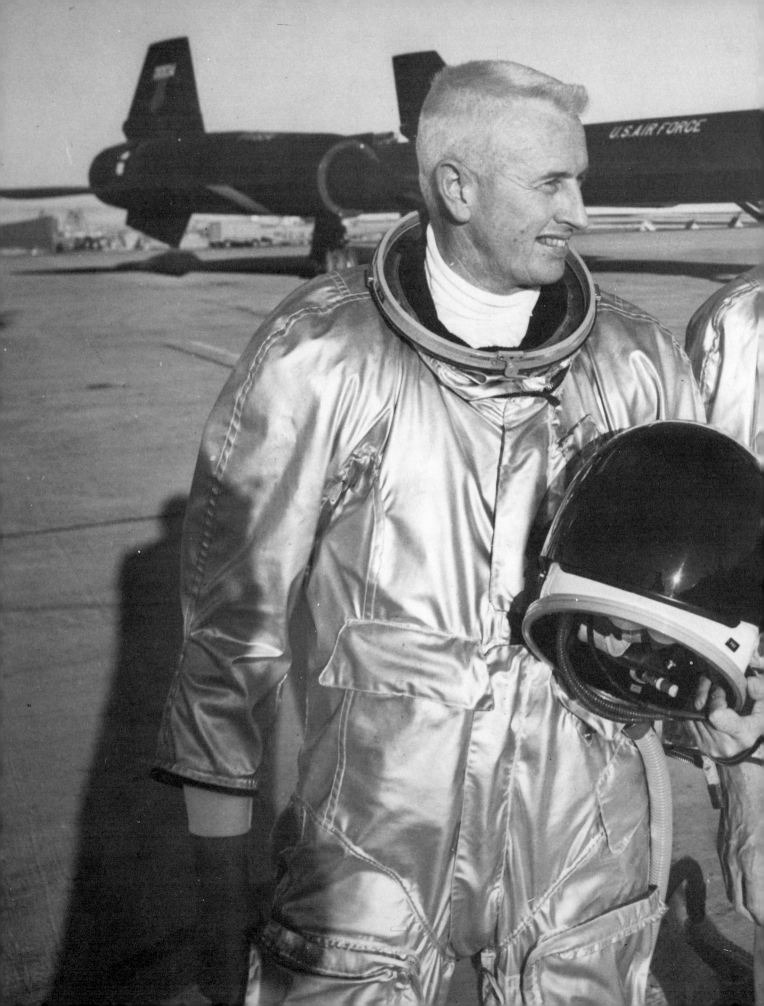

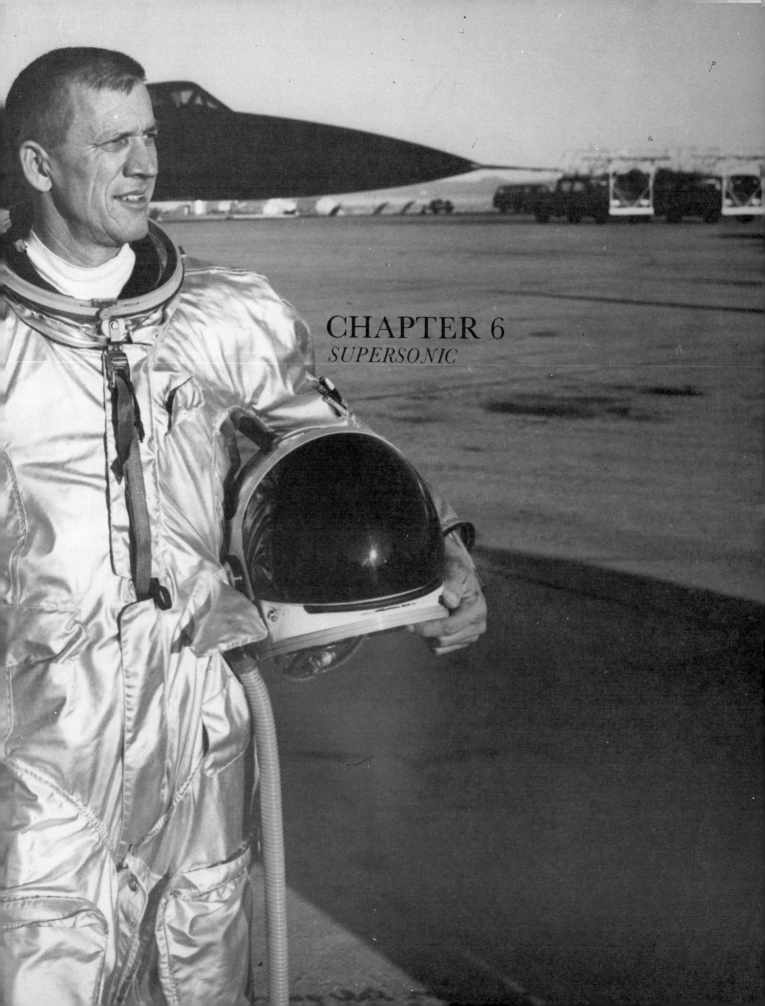

CHAPTER 6
SUPERSONIC

Post-war euphoria was not, unfortunately, to last long. Open hostilities had ceased but Cold-War aggressions rumbled away menacingly like subterranean tremors heralding an earthquake. Russia's development of the atomic bomb in 1949 kept the Western world on its toes, sustaining the momentum of wartime aeronautical developments. There was no time for the West to sit back and rest on its laurels for the arms race was well under way. The West had not only to keep abreast of its competitors but also be in a state of constant readiness in case of attack. Wars such as the ones in Korea in 1950, in Malaya during the fifties, Suez in 1956 and Vietnam from 1956 to 1974 brought home the real possibility of a third world war.

An idea of the astounding rate of progress in the field of aviation during the post-war years can be seen by a comparison of world speed records. In 1946 a Gloster Meteor F.Mk4 established a record of 615 mph. This record was broken repeatedly until in 1968 it passed to a North American X-15 which attained the awesome speed of 4,534 mph. Progress of this sort can be attributed largely to innovations in the fields of aircraft propulsion, aerodynamics and airframe construction, to the development of thin swept-back wings, after-burners and heat-resistant alloys of elements such as titanium.

In 1947 Major Charles E. Yeager of the USAF was the first to break the challenging sound barrier in level flight when he flew the rocket-powered Bell X1 at over 760 mph. The supersonic era had dawned. Only the short-sightedness of politicians or the physiological limitations of the human body could inhibit these tremendous aeronautical advances. Jet aircraft were first seen, in relatively small numbers, towards the end of World War II. By the early fifties Meteors, Vampires and Canberras were used by many squadrons. The V-bomber force with Valiants, Victors and Vulcans reigned supreme from the mid-fifties to the mid-sixties. Britain's first supersonic fighter/interceptor was the English Electric Lightning. Introduced in 1960, this aircraft can climb to 50,000 ft in one minute and fly at 1,500 mph at 40,000 ft. It is not difficult to appreciate the great strains a Lightning pilot has to undergo, especially when one compares the performance of the Lightning with the performance of a Spitfire Mk IX of 1942. The latter's maximum speed was 415 mph and it took over eight minutes to reach 30,000 ft. At the speeds at which a Lightning can travel there is little time for seeing, recognising and avoiding another aircraft, a matter of a second or so. Many high-performance aircraft can withstand 'G' forces far beyond the tolerance of man and fly at altitudes that would kill a man within seconds if he were not well protected. Man has devised aircraft that can hurtle through the hostile environment of the stratosphere at several times the speed of sound, yet in several thousand years man himself, his faculties and reactions, have changed little. Can he withstand the great physical stresses that may be imposed on him, is he mentally capable of coping with the complexities of supersonic flight under differing conditions? It is unlikely that his reactions when flying a Lightning at 1,000 mph could ever be ten times quicker than when driving a car at 100 mph.

Pressurisation

Thanks largely to the work in the field of aviation medicine the human aspects of flight have at last been recognised as of major importance and the pilot's stresses and strains handled with as much diligence as those of the aircraft; for however advanced an aircraft may be, it can be flown only within the limits of the pilot's tolerance. This tolerance can be raised artificially, by the aircraft engineer and the flying-clothing designer.

The engineer's main contribution is the pressurisation and conditioning of cockpits and cabins. This helps to normalise conditions by alleviating, if not eliminating, hypoxia, dysbarism and cold, by increasing comfort and so reducing fatigue. Modern jet aircraft, both civil and military, need to fly in the thinner air of the upper atmosphere to enable them to fly economically at greater speeds. All these aircraft are therefore pressurised.

Pressurised aircraft were being introduced during the last war and in the post-war era are quite common. By increasing the pressure inside an aircraft as it climbs to altitude, an environment more akin to that on earth is being simulated. It would obviously be ideal to be able to pressurise an aircraft to sea-level pressure at whatever height it is flying, but at altitude to compensate fully for the difference between cabin pressure and outside air pressure would necessitate considerable strengthening of the fuselage, thereby increasing the weight of the aircraft. The design of an aircraft always involves compromise, and the problem of pressurisation is no exception.

A high pressure differential is required for civil airliners so that when the aircraft is flying at 40,000 ft the cabin altitude is the equivalent of only 8,000 ft. Thus, unless an emergency occurs, passengers have no need to use oxygen masks. On the other hand a low pressure differential is used for most military aircraft since failure of pressure as a result of enemy action is always a hazard. If cabin pressure fails, the higher the pressure differential, the less likely are one's chances of escape, or survival. Military high-altitude aircraft maintain a pressure differential of only $3\frac{1}{2}$ lb/in² as opposed to the civil airliners' $8\frac{1}{4}$ lb/in². Some long-range bomber aircraft have a 'cruise setting' of 9 lb/in² to reduce fatigue on long journeys, but a 'combat setting' of a much lower pressure differential when action may be expected; the effect being that a B52, for example, can fly at 60,000 ft with the much more comfortable cabin altitude of 13,500 ft.

However, if for some reason cabin pressure is lost, the situation becomes far from ideal. The rate of decompression is critical and depends on many factors including the pressure differential at the time, the size of the hole in the airframe, the volume that is depressurised and whether flood-flow air supplies are available. In the event of such an accident military airmen usually have a better chance of survival than the airline pilot and his passengers since they can dive their aircraft faster to a lower and safer altitude, and they will in any case be wearing oxygen masks and protective pressure clothing to suit the operating mode. They may also have the opportunity to abandon their aircraft by ejecting themselves if control of the aircraft is lost. We shall be discussing these points later in the chapter.

Shirt-sleeve flying in a Boeing 707. This type of headset is worn by both airline and private pilots.

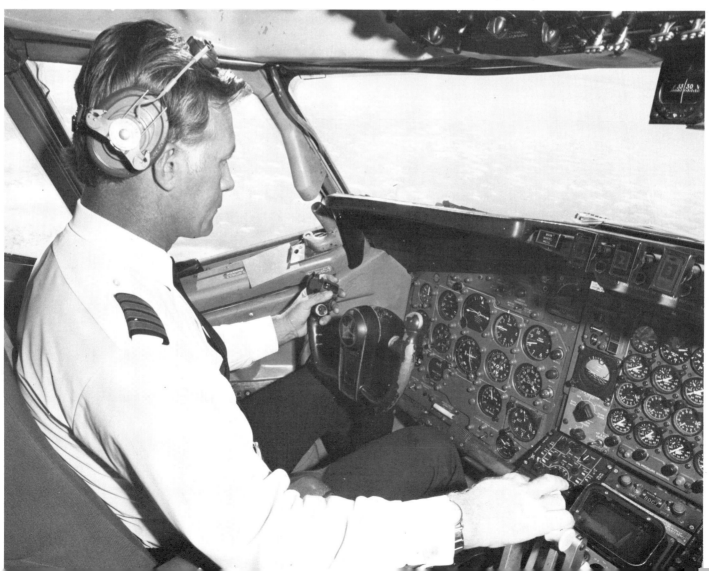

If cabin pressure is lost in a civil airliner an emergency descent has to be carried out as quickly as possible. If the structure of the aircraft has been damaged the aircraft may be unable to withstand the strains of a rapid descent and may break up, as in the case of the Comet disasters. The average cruising altitude of most airliners is about 33,000ft, and at this height a person in a decompressed aircraft would lose consciousness in probably less than a minute. Yet an emergency descent from this altitude to 14,000ft may take two minutes. The individual oxygen supplies above each seat would have to be used immediately and, most important of all, the pilot would have to go on to his emergency oxygen supply as soon as he had initiated the emergency descent. These problems are exaggerated with supersonic aircraft such as Concorde and the Tu144 which fly at 60,000–70,000ft. If cabin pressure is lost at over 40,000ft, even with oxygen, one would have less than thirty seconds of useful consciousness, and at 63,000ft the body fluids boil. Pressurisation failure, therefore, clearly presents a major hazard. However, a high degree of protection has been achieved in Concorde by the incorporation of such features as small windows and multiple high-capacity air supplies (flood flow) so that, except in the event of a major catastrophe, a cabin altitude of 25,000ft can be maintained and life sustained by the use of emergency oxygen equipment until lower altitudes are reached. Little does a businessman realise as he climbs nonchalantly into Concorde wearing his best pin-striped suit that he will be hurtled through a totally hostile atmosphere where military pilots fly dressed like spacemen.

The aircraft engineer has done his bit to normalise conditions in flight by providing pressurisation. It is only on very rare occasions in civil flying that this sytem fails, but military aircraft, by the very nature of their role, are more vulnerable. Enemy action may cause loss of cabin pressure and, furthermore, a pilot may be forced to abandon his aircraft if for one reason or another he is unable to maintain control. Therefore, although most military aircraft are pressurised, there is always the possibility of things going wrong, and so there is a need for a back-up system, which is provided by specialised flying clothing.

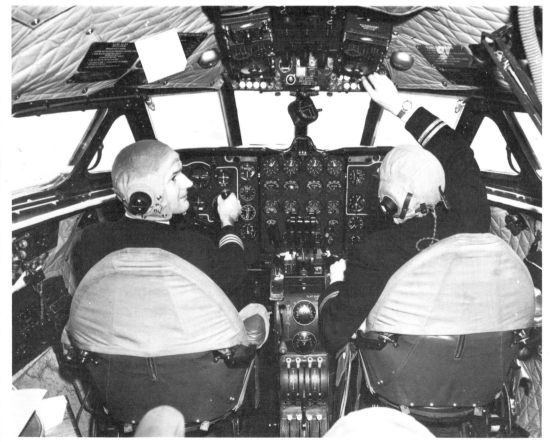

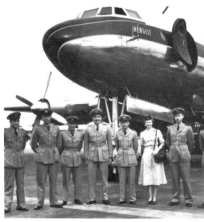

A Comet flightdeck. The pilots are weari[ng] RAF Type E wired helments.

The BOAC aircrew of a Handley Pa[ge] Hermes, early 50's. They are continuing t[he] Imperial Airways tradition of wearin[g] tropical khaki clothing.

The majority of military aircraft tend to operate at altitudes where oxygen is required, but rarely under pressure. Even high-performance aircraft that have considerable ceilings are required in modern warfare to fly very low in order to dodge enemy radar. It is mainly the reconnaissance/spy plane, the long-range bomber aircraft and the interceptor that operate at altitudes above 40,000 ft where pressure-breathing is necessary. In all military aircraft whose cabin altitude will exceed 8,000 ft, oxygen is routinely breathed to prevent any loss in aircrew performance. Up to 50,000 ft protection can be maintained by the use of an oronasal mask with a positive pressure of oxygen supplied to the mask to maintain the correct oxygen proportions in the blood stream. At altitudes above 50,000 ft this positive-pressure level has to be increased beyond the limits which can be sustained by the human frame and positive-pressure garments have to be worn which apply an equal pressure to the outside of the body to oppose the internal pressure. The function of breathing with increased pressure levels in the body is known as pressure-breathing.

During World War II the Economiser system of oxygen delivery was used. The flow of oxygen was determined by a manually set regulator, and air for dilution at lower altitudes was admitted through a valve in the side of the mask. Soon after the war the Demand System was introduced. With this system the amount of oxygen delivered is controlled automatically by the regulator. An aneroid capsule gives the right mix of air, which is admitted at the regulator instead of at the mask, thus reducing the possibility of water vapour freezing in the mask and causing a failure of the system. This system

BEA Stewardesses through the ages. From left to right, 1947, 1954, 1960, 1967.

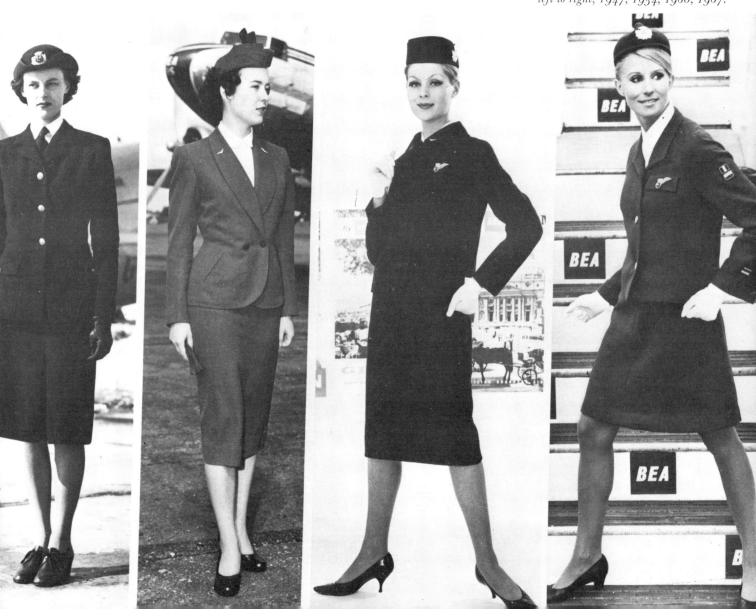

allows for changing rates of respiration and can also be used for pressure-breathing. A well-sealed oxygen mask is vital, since the demand valve does not operate until the mask pressure falls below that of the environment. A well-sealed mask further reduces the risk of freezing and minimises displacement by radial acceleration or ejection blast. The G and H Type masks were used shortly after the war but the Type J mask was the first to be used by the RAF with a demand system. Introduced in about 1951 it was superseded by the American A13A series made of green moulded rubber and by the P and Q series in the sixties. These masks all have a reflected edge which, acting as an efficient seal against the face, prevents leakage. The black P and Q Type masks have a chain-tensioned toggle device which can be quickly tightened for pressure-breathing up to 56,000 ft.

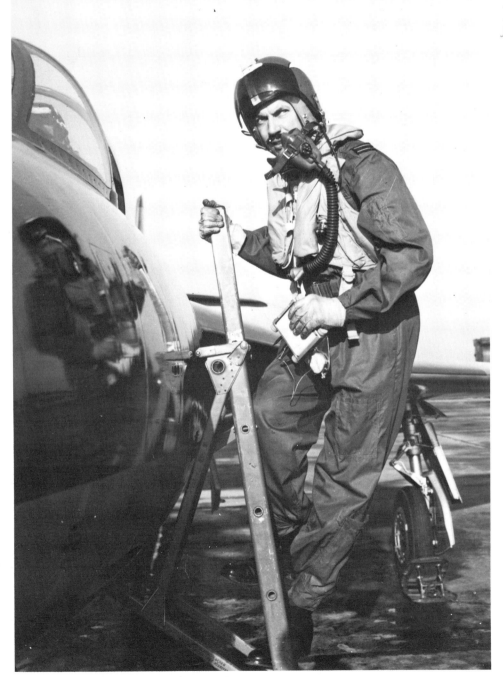

A pilot climbing into his Hunter wearing Mk 1A Bone Dome, Type G helmet a... A-13A mask with the early pattern gr... flying overalls. Boscombe Down, 1957.

A pilot wearing a Mk 1A Bo... Dome, Type G helmet and 'P' Ty... mask. The P and Q Type Mas... are identical in design and dif... only in size of face piece, the ... Type being the smaller.

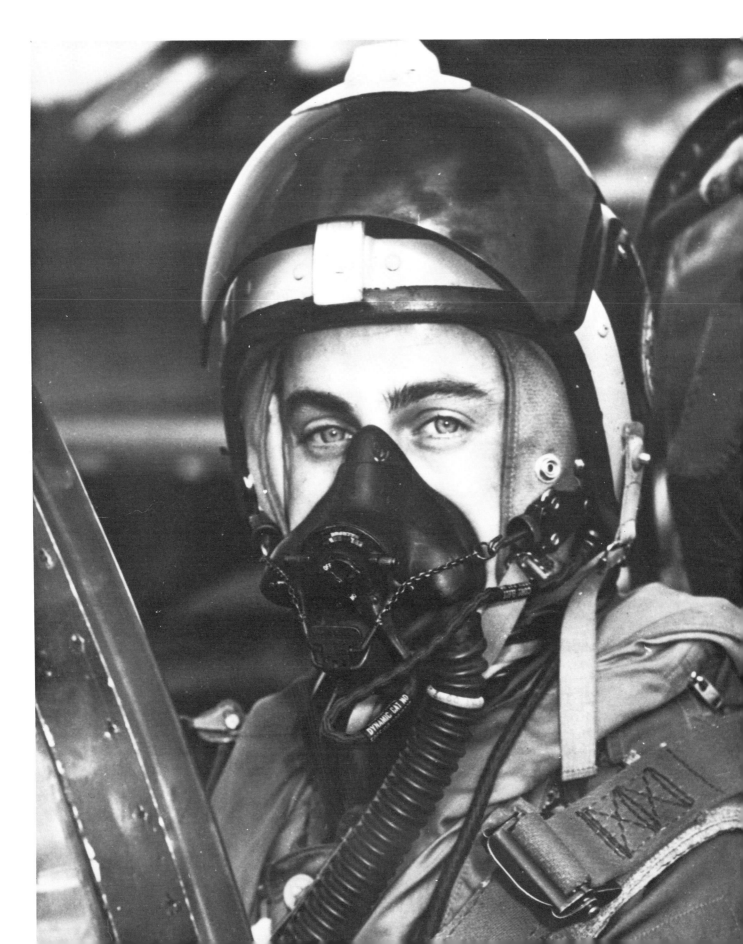

Regulators for the demand system were originally mounted in the airframe. America developed a mask-mounted 100-per-cent demand regulator which eliminated the flow-resistance of the connecting hose. In the 1960s Britain introduced a man-mounted miniature regulator which is used in the Phantom, Harrier, Nimrod and Jaguar, but recent arguments propose a return to the seat-mounted regulator which is larger, more robust and less likely to be damaged by rough handling. Furthermore, it is cheaper to provide one regulator per aircraft than one per man. A demand regulator incorporating a stand-by regulator has been introduced for long-range and high-altitude aircraft so that flight can be continued if the main regulator fails. This sophisticated system is in use in the Jaguar and will be used in the Tornado and Hawk. Demand systems provide air increasingly enriched by oxygen up to 30,000ft, pure oxygen above 30,000ft and automatic pressure-breathing from 40,000 to 70,000ft.

Since cabin altitudes are reduced by pressurisation, oxygen equipment is usually required only at maximum altitudes, unless the aircraft has a low pressure differential. But if pressurisation fails, oxygen equipment must be immediately to hand. For example, a Boeing B52 Stratofortress flying at 35,000ft will have a cabin altitude of only 8,000ft; the crew will therefore not be using oxygen. But if the cabin pressure failed they would lose consciousness within half a minute without oxygen. When flying at these altitudes the masks should always be readily available in case of decompression. If pressurisation is lost above 45,000ft, even when pure unpressurised oxygen is being breathed, the time of useful consciousness is a matter of a minute or so, since the barometric pressure is inadequate to maintain an oxygen pressure in the lungs sufficient to ensure satisfactory oxygenation of the blood. At these altitudes a back-up pressure system is required.

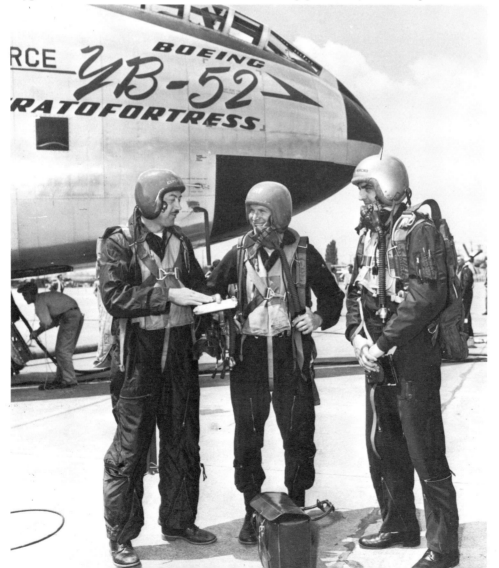

B-52 aircrew wearing standard American flying clothing, including the A-13A oxygen mask. A. M. "Tex" Johnston, then B-52 test pilot, is on the left.

Pressurisation and clothing

Pressure suits were developed during the thirties for high-altitude record-breaking attempts. Once pressure cabins had been introduced, pressure suits were necessary only as a secondary system against loss of cabin pressurisation, a safeguard introduced first of all by Germany. Pressurisation of the whole man by enclosing him entirely in an air-tight suit is obviously the ideal insurance against loss of cabin pressure at great altitude, but in practice full-pressure clothing is heavy, bulky, hot and inflexible. The American Navy did much work in the development of a practical full-pressure suit in the fifties, and in 1959 produced a lightweight version known as the A/P22S-3. A more advanced model, the A/P22S-2, the precursor of the space suit, was used in the X15 project, and is used in long-range, high-altitude aircraft such as the Lockheed SR71 (Blackbird) which is reputed to cruise at well over 2,000 mph at heights of up to 85,000 ft. With the development in the sixties of long-range reconnaissance/spy planes the use of a full-pressure suit ensured that, in the event of loss of cabin pressure at high altitude, the mission could be completed; thus they are often known as 'mission-completion suits'. The full-pressure suit protects the pilot not only against anoxia but also against the intense cold of altitude.

The crew of the SR-71, the Blackbird. They are wearing a silver coloured Nomex outer suit over an olive green full pressure suit which is effective at altitudes in excess of 100,000 feet. A plain white outer suit has recently been introduced which has improved flame resistance. Rubber and nylon in the pressure suit tends to melt, run and stick—hence the Nomex outer garment.

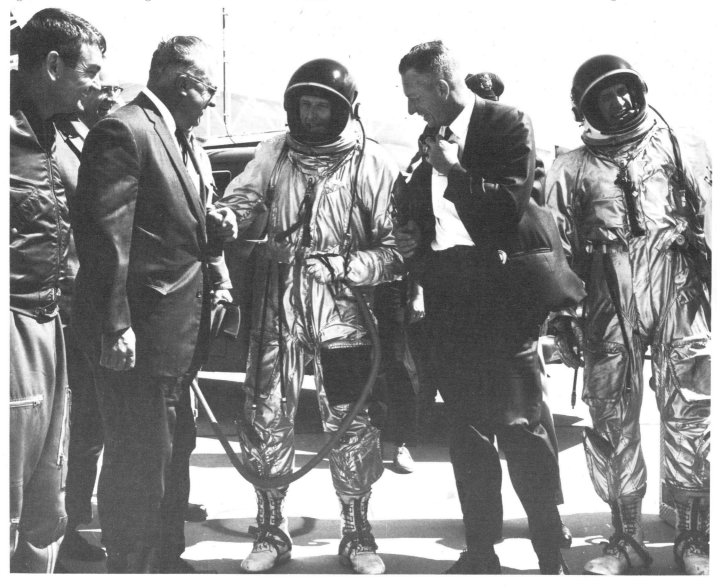

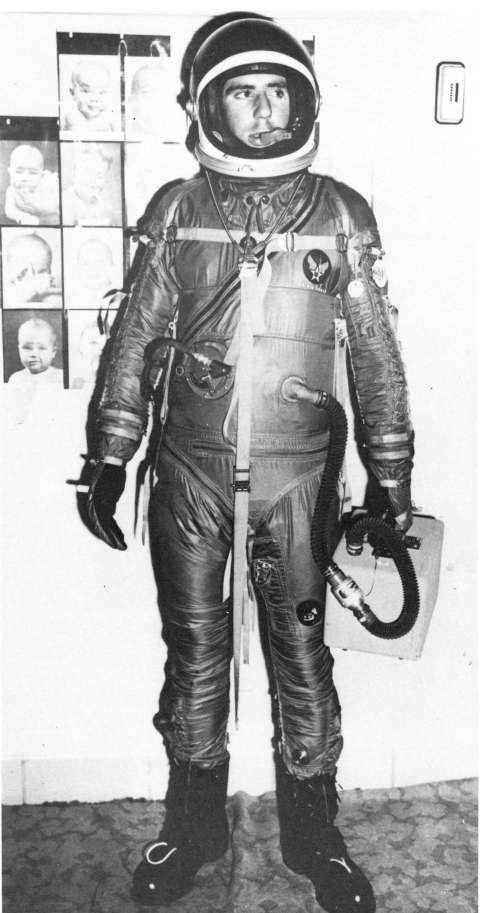

The United States Air Force AP 22S-
full pressure suit, which was developed i
the late 1950's from the US Navy/B. F
Goodrich Mk IV full pressure suit. I
combines high altitude protection with sur
vival protection for the pilot, should he b
forced to land or abandon his aircraft i
Polar regions or cold water.

A more welcome alternative to the uncomfortable and unwieldy full-pressure suit is the partial-pressure suit or 'get-me-down suit'. Like the full-pressure suit it is worn uninflated but is inflated automatically by an aneroid-controlled regulator in the event of decompression above 40,000 ft. As its name implies, it is essentially a back-up pressurisation system used in the event of an emergency to facilitate a rapid controlled descent to safer altitudes. It provides short-term as opposed to the long-term protection of a full-pressure suit and is used on a much wider scale than the full-pressure suit.

There are two methods of partial pressurisation in use. The one that was developed in America in the late forties, the T1 suit, applied a system of mechanical counter-pressure to the body, a method originally used for anti-'G' protection. The suit was a close-fitting garment made of nylon-cotton twill with small inflatable tubes or capstans which ran across the pilot's back and down the outer sides of both arms and legs and were attached to the suit by crossing tapes. The tapes tightened when the capstans were inflated, making the suit skin-tight and perfectly counterbalancing the pressure inside the pilot's lungs. This suit, which included anti-'G' protection, was used in X1 supersonic flights of 1948 and could provide protection at 100,000 ft for six minutes. Later models such as the MC3A incorporate a torso bladder which enables the pilot to remain at 100,000 ft for over an hour. This suit was used in the U2 spy plane programme. Even when uninflated these suits had to be skin-tight and were very hot to wear. A pilot would lose from four to five pounds from perspiring during prolonged flights in the upper atmosphere; little wonder that they were sometimes referred to as 'sweat suits'. An equally important part of altitude suit assembly is the high-pressure oxygen helmet. The MA2 helmet has a cloth neckpiece which extends down inside the suit providing a satisfactory seal for high breathing pressures. Pressure clothing is always worn by military flying personnel when altitudes of 50,000 ft are to be exceeded.

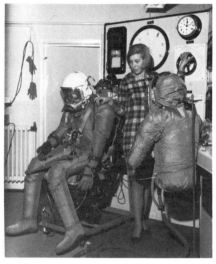

Experimental work at the Institute of Aviation Medicine, 1963.

Herman "Fish" Salmon, former Chief Test Pilot for Lockheed, wearing a Capstan partial pressure suit, standing by his Starfighter.

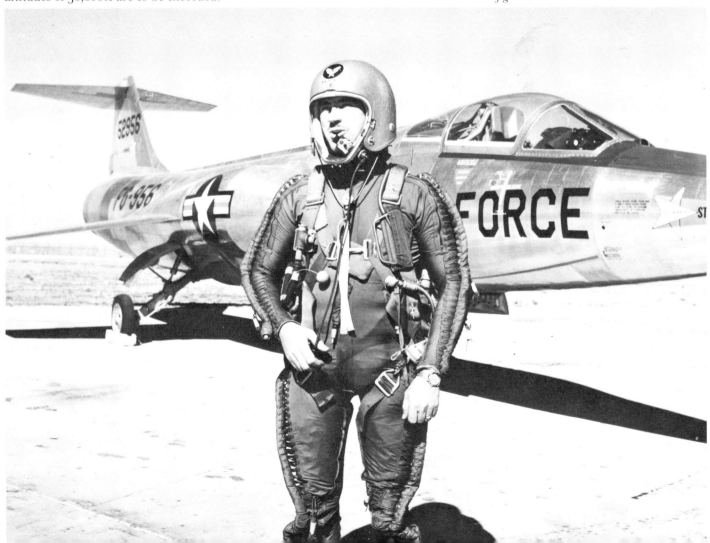

Britain also developed a practical full-pressure suit after the war but concentrated much more on partial pressurisation. The full-pressure suit was not introduced because the V-bomber operational mode was changing. The V-bombers, introduced in the mid-fifties, were conceived as high-altitude bomber and reconnaissance aircraft, but the appearance in the late fifties of surface-to-air missiles posed a clear threat to high-altitude operations and invalidated the original V-bomber concept. V-bombers now dashed across the tree tops to avoid enemy radar. Full-pressure, mission-completion suits were therefore not required. In conjunction with the American Aid Programme in the early fifties, when Britain was supplied with F86 Sabres she adopted the American capstan partial-pressure suit for a few years, but simultaneously was designing her own partial- pressure waistcoat, which was based on a Canadian example of the 1940s. Instead of applying counter-pressure to the body mechanically by means of small inflated tubes the pressure waistcoat consisted of two layers of fabric which were rubberised on the inside, and the

Boeing pilots having their partial pressur equipment tested before a flight in a B-52.

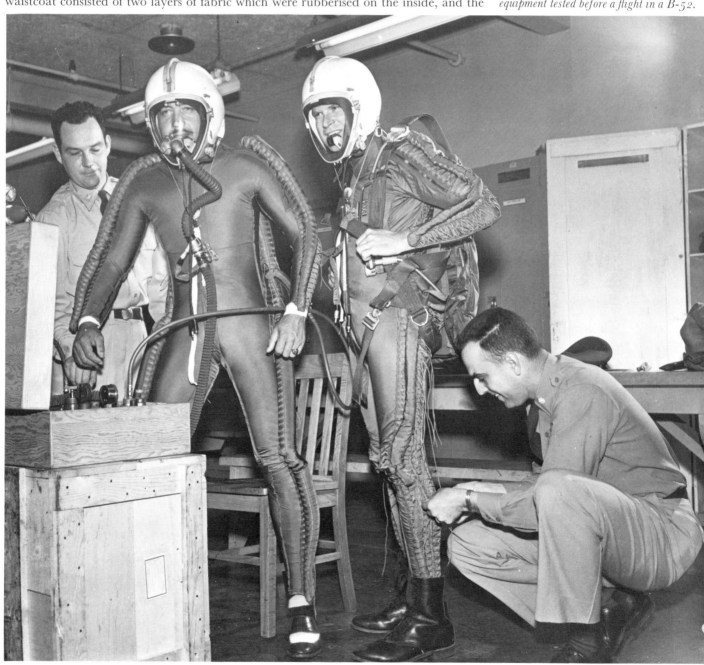

whole waistcoat was inflated to provide counter-pressure to the body. The waistcoat was zipped up the front and laced up the back to fit the wearer. It was used with the Type J or Type M, pressure-demand oxygen mask which received unpressurised oxygen up to 35,000 ft and pressurised oxygen from 35,000 to 43,000 ft. This was the maximum altitude attainable for an indefinite period, although for limited periods it provided protection up to 48,000 ft. These waistcoats were used in early Hunters, Javelins, the Canberra PR9, V-bombers and the Lightning. Compared to contemporary American partial-pressure equipment, the British pressure waistcoat was relatively ineffective. In 1958, however, a pressure jerkin was introduced which covered the chest, trunk and upper thighs and proved much more successful. Like the waistcoat, it operated on an inflatable bladder principle. It was worn with anti-'G' trousers, an air-ventilated suit and a partial-pressure helmet. Unlike an ordinary bone-dome or anti-buffet helmet, the partial-pressure helmet introduced in 1956 encloses the whole head and neck and pressurises a considerable area of the head and neck as well as the cheeks and floor of the mouth. It has an integral pressure-breathing mask and a barometrically operated visor which clamps automatically into place to provide an oxygen-tight unit in the event of an emergency at high altitude. The partial-pressure helmet and pressure-jerkin oxygen supply are interconnected so that the external and internal pressures are equal. A special barathea battledress with elastic-waisted trousers was introduced for wear over the partial-pressure assembly.

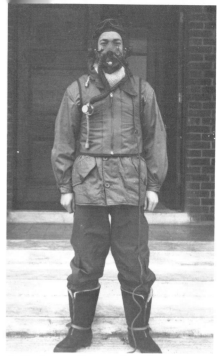

A Canberra pilot wearing the early style Pressure Waistcoat and Type J mask, Type C helmet, Mk VIII goggles and 1941 Pattern boots.

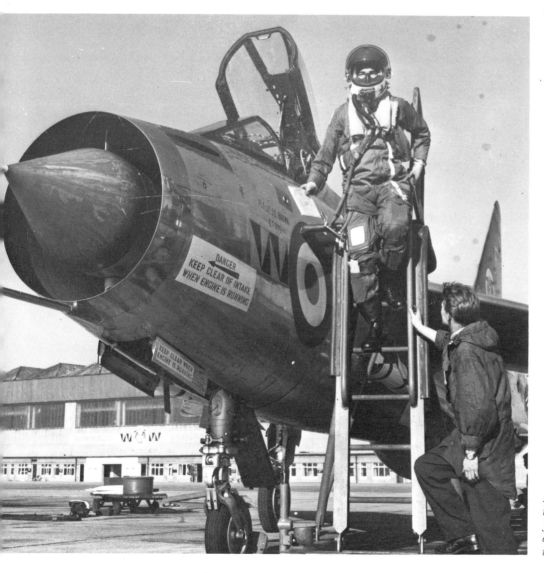

A Lightning pilot from Coltishall in 1963 in a Partial Pressure helmet and Pressure Jerkin. He is wearing 1952 Pattern boots and the blue/grey flying suit commonly worn in the late 50's and early 1960's.

143

Protection for longer periods is provided by increased body coverage. Thus a pilot wearing a partial-pressure helmet, a pressure jerkin with sleeves and anti-'G' trousers will be afforded greater protection than one who simply has a pressure-demand mask, a pressure jerkin without sleeves and anti-'G' trousers. A pilot in the early sixties would often have had innumerable items of flying clothing to put on and a multitude of connections to make once he was in his aircraft. But in recent years there has been a trend to integrate clothing in an attempt to simplify matters. In 1966 a combined partial-pressure and anti-'G' flying suit was introduced, followed a year later by a combined partial-pressure anti-'G' and air-ventilated suit in an olive-drab colour known as Coverall, High-Altitude, Anti-'G', Ventilated, which is used today for high-altitude flying. However, although military aircraft are pressurised to be able to fly at great heights and their pilots are given a protective back-up system in case of loss of cabin pressure, they must at all costs be able to dodge the enemy's radar, and this involves flying at a height of only a few hundred feet. Thus pressure clothing does not have such a widespread role to play as in former years. Even the long-range, high-altitude spy planes have largely been superseded by reconnaissance satellites.

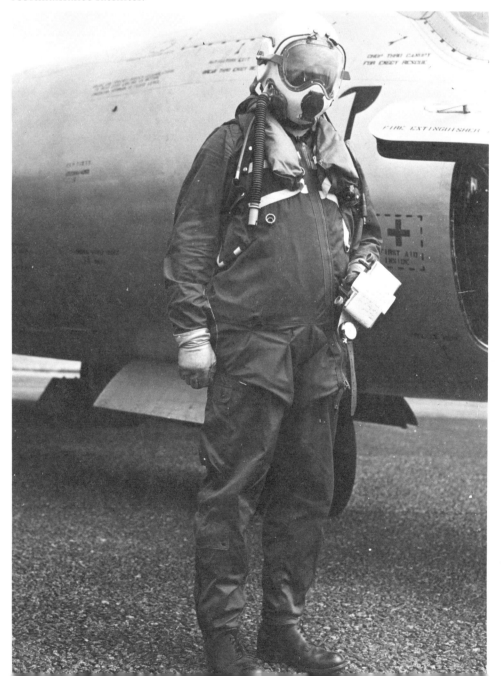

Wing Commander R. P. Beamont in his pressure clothing after flying the Canberra Mk 9. 1956. The life preserver is built into the Pressure Jerkin. The central flap in the helmet below the visor facilities eating and drinking.

Since the introduction of jet aircraft, operating speeds have risen so dramatically that, in the event of an emergency, aircrews can no longer clamber out of the cockpit and jump to safety. They would almost certainly be dashed against the fuselage by the vicious slip-stream or become entangled in the tailplane if they were able to get out at all; although it should be mentioned that crew members sitting in the rear of such aircraft as the Vulcan do not have assisted escape and have to leave the aircraft through hatches or doors. Germany pioneered the field of assisted escape in the early forties but within a few years Britain took the lead.

A Harrier pilot wearing the summer Aircrew Equipment Assembly strapped into his Martin-Baker ejection seat. He is wearing a Protective Helmet Mk 2A and a P Type mask. Note the man-mounted oxygen regulator and the leg restraint garters.

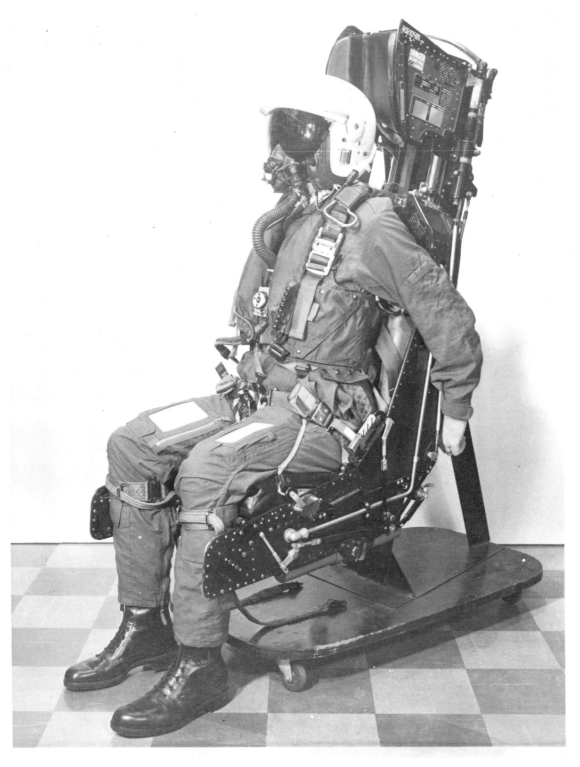

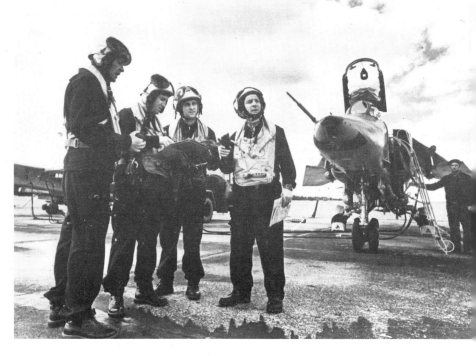

A Russian Mikoyan MiG-23 and crew.

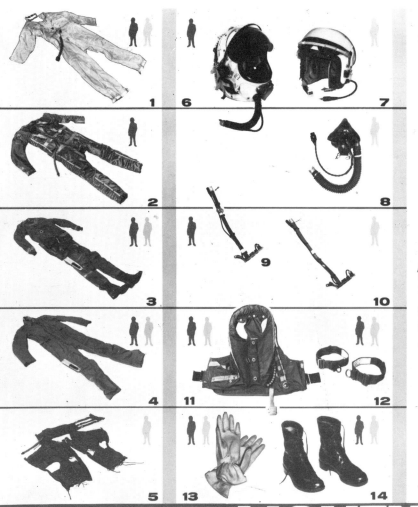

ITEM NO.	SECTION REF. NO.	DESCRIPTION
1	22C 1856 - 1911	AIR VENTILATED SUIT Mk. 2
2	22C 2708 - 2717	COMBINED PRESSURE ANTI-G SU
3	22C 2718 - 2725	IMMERSION SUIT Mk. 8
4	22C 2746 - 2754	L WEIGHT FLYING SUIT Mk.8
5		
6	22C 2093 - 2,115	PARTIAL PRESSURE HELMET BV type
7		
8		
9	6G 1249	PRESSURE JERKIN HOSE assy. Mk
10		
11	22C 2744	JACKET LIFESAVING Mk. 9B
12	22C 2024	GARTERS (leg restraint) Q.R.
13	22C 1445 - 45	GLOVES water resistant Mk.2
14	22C 2778 - 2744	BOOTS FLYING (new pattern)

NOTES...

1. For further details of clothing and connectors refer to the relevant chapter of AP 1182 VOL.1 BK. 2 or LIGHTNING M AEA schedule.

2. All aircrew must receive indoctrination training before flying with this equipment. For limitations of equipment refer to Pilo Notes, AP 4700c - P.N. pt.1. chapter 12. para.

ITEM NO.	SECTION REF. NO.	DESCRIPTION
1	22C 1856 - 1911	AIR VENTILATED SUIT Mk. 2A
2		
3	22C 2718 - 2725	IMMERSION SUIT Mk. 8
4	22C 2746 - 2754	L WEIGHT FLYING SUIT Mk.
5	22C 1911 - 1944	ANTI-G SUIT Mk. 5A
6		
7	22C 2467 - 2469 & 2711	PROTECTIVE HELMET Mk. 2A
8	6C 2517 & 2305	OXYGEN MASK (type P2A or Q2A
9		
10	6C 2073	OXYGEN MASK HOSE ASSY. Mk
11	22C 2744	JACKET LIFESAVING Mk. 9B
12	22C 2024	GARTERS (leg restraint) Q.R.
13	22C 1440 - 45	GLOVES—water resistant Mk.2
14	22C 2778 - 2744	BOOTS FLYING (new pattern)

AIRCREW EQUIPMENT ASSEMBLIES **LIGHTNING** Mk 3

ML AVIATION CO. LTD.

WHITE WALTHAM AERODROME

MAIDENHEAD BERKSHIRE ENG

DRG NO P 1384   DATE 16.10

DRAWN I.R.B.   CHECKED F.L

In 1944 Mr (now Sir) James Martin, Managing Director of Martin-Baker Aircraft Company, was approached by the then Ministry of Aircraft Production to see if he could produce a means of assisted escape for fighter pilots. He designed a seat which, by means of an explosive charge, was ejected from the aircraft with the occupant sitting in it. After ejection the pilot would unharness himself from the seat and pull the parachute rip-cord in the usual way. The Martin-Baker Mk1 ejection seat proved a great success, saving many lives. However, to insure against the possibility of a pilot losing consciousness on ejection and thereafter being unable to detach himself from the seat and open the 'chute, an ejection seat was introduced in the early 1950s in which the whole sequence of events operated automatically. The development of ejection or 'bang' seats has kept pace with the increased performance of aircraft and can virtually guarantee the pilot's safety in almost all aspects of flight. The main problem has been successful assisted escape at low altitude and speed. A very high proportion of accidents occur on take-off

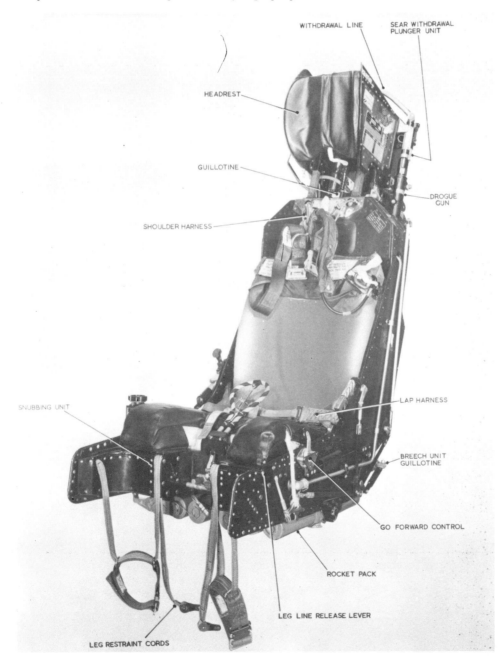

WITHDRAWAL LINE
SEAR WITHDRAWAL PLUNGER UNIT
HEADREST
GUILLOTINE
DROGUE GUN
SHOULDER HARNESS
LAP HARNESS
SNUBBING UNIT
BREECH UNIT GUILLOTINE
GO FORWARD CONTROL
ROCKET PACK
LEG LINE RELEASE LEVER
LEG RESTRAINT CORDS

A Martin-Baker Type 9A Mk 2 ejection seat.

or landing, and assisted escape at these levels demands that the pilot be ejected to at least two hundred feet so that the parachute canopy has time to open fully. In 1962, in preference to the explosive charge, a rocket pack was installed in the seat, this prolongs the thrust without subjecting the pilot to any excessive acceleration. The new method proved especially successful when ejecting from aircraft with high fins such as the Javelin or the V-bombers and when ejecting from VTOL aircraft such as the Harrier, which has a very high sink-rate and no forward speed if the engine fails on take-off or landing.

Only one per cent of assisted escapes occur above 30,000 ft, but if a pilot is forced to bale out at any great altitude, especially if he is travelling at supersonic speed, his return to earth is unlikely to be a pleasant one. When subjected to supersonic blast a man may be stripped of his helmet, oxygen mask and gloves and although there are leg restraint garters on all ejection seats neither the arms nor the head are restrained. Arm restraint is being introduced along with a double form of leg restraint in the Tornado, securing the lower legs and the thighs. Hypoxia would result from loss of oxygen mask at altitude and large quantities of air would be forced into a man's stomach and lungs. Loss of bone-dome and visor may result in a badly bruised or lacerated face and torn eyelids. However, the chances of being seriously injured are greatly reduced if correct procedures are followed. Once the man has ejected, a drogue stabilises the seat to prevent tumbling and spinning. After a predetermined delay (ususally between 1·5 and 2·25 secs) the seat and man automatically separate and the main parachute deploys. However, if an incident occurs above 10,000 ft (or any other pre-selected height) the sequence just described is modified in that the man and the seat do not automatically separate until the pre-selected height has been reached. An emergency oxygen supply is used during the descent until seat/man separation.

Hunter pilots of 257 Squadron in the ear. 1950's wearing the Type G helmet and Mk Bone Dome with a separate visor attached t an elasticated strap. Note the Squadro markings painted on the Bone Domes. The are also wearing A-13A masks, yellow li, preservers and grey flying overalls.

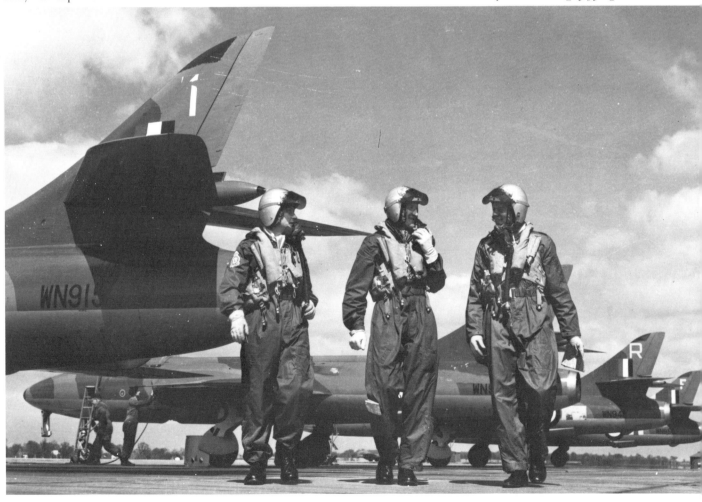

The introduction of aircraft ejection has demanded certain adjustments and innovations in the field of flying clothing, the most notable of which is the bone-dome. The bone-dome, bone-box or brain bucket is officially known as an anti-buffet helmet or Helmet, Flying, Protective. It was first used in America in about 1950 where it was known as a Lombard helmet. Originally designed for protection against buffeting and in the event of a crash, it was regarded with reserve by British authorities who felt that it would impose an unwarranted load on the wearer's neck during high-'G' manoeuvres. However, in 1952 the RAF issued a requirement for a helmet providing not only protection against crash impact and against the buffeting which frequently occurs during high-speed, low-level flight, but also protection during ejection. The 2nd TAF was being issued with Sabres, whose ejection seats were trigger-fired from the seat arm-rest rather than by the normal British method of pulling down a face-protection blind. It was therefore vital that the pilot's face and head be fully protected from the devastating wind-blast experienced with high-speed ejection. The face-blind firing handle used on all aircraft fitted with British-designed ejection seats had many advantages. Because the pilot had to reach above his head to pull the blind it ensured that he was sitting in a safe, upright position and, further-more, it protected the face and head from wind-blast. However, if the aircraft was in a tight manoeuvre where high positive 'G' forces were applied it was often impossible for the pilot to reach the blind at all. Seat-pan firing handles have therefore been fitted to many seats as an alternative to the face-blind handle, the bone-dome and visor providing the only protection against wind-blast if the seat-actuator is used. The latest seats have only the seat-pan firing handle. Bone-domes also protect the head if the cockpit canopy release mechanism fails and the pilot is ejected straight through the canopy. A pilot may even choose to eject through the canopy if he is near ground level where every split second counts.

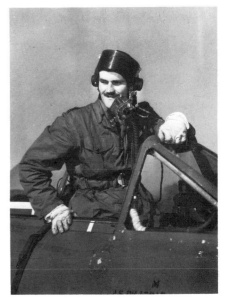

Sqn. Ldr. D. H. Seaton, DFC, former O.C. No 11 Squadron, in his Venom. He is wearing the Type C helmet with Mk 1 visor attached and Type J oxygen mask.

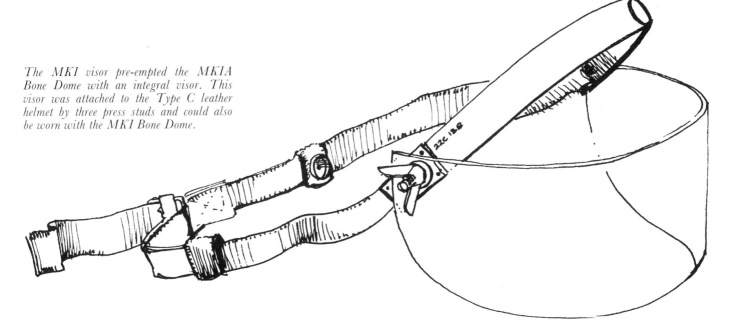

The MKI visor pre-empted the MKIA Bone Dome with an integral visor. This visor was attached to the Type C leather helmet by three press studs and could also be worn with the MKI Bone Dome.

The RAF's Mk I protective helmet was worn with goggles or a separate visor over a Type G inner helmet which incorporated the earphones; the Mk IA had an anti-glare visor attached by a central track onto the bone-dome. The Mk 2A combined the features of the Mk IA and Type G helmets and had a surface-dyed, anti-blast and glare visor which locked automatically on ejection. The visor suffered easily from scratch damage and had to be treated with care. The Mks 3A and 3B were for aircraft without ejection seats and had the Mk IA helmet-type glare visor attached on a central track. The Mk 4A super sedes all other designs and is for the use of all aircrew operating in high- or low-altitude aircraft, with or without ejection seats. This helmet is fitted with a double visor system.

Physiological problems

Another item of aircrew equipment that was redesigned in the mid-1960s to withstand ejection wind-blast is the life-jacket or life-preserver. The Terylene waistcoat is olive-drab in colour. A blast-proof pouch covering the inflatable stole ensures a very compact design. After ejection the beaded operating handle is pulled, the pouch is opened and the fluorescent, orange-coloured nylon stole inflated instantly from a CO_2 cyclinder. Search and rescue aids are positioned in pockets. A life-preserver has been designed which inflates automatically on immersion in water – a valuable piece of equipment to airmen who are incapacitated on ejection. Some life-preservers and the torso parachute harness are integrated. Life-preservers are fastened by metal closure plates rather than buttons when the man-mounted oxygen regulator is used.

One of the most common injuries suffered on ejection is crushed vertebrae. If the man is not sitting upright and his harness has not been adjusted correctly his spine can be damaged by the large 'G' forces experienced both on ejection and when the parachute opens. Effective body restraint is vital to prevent body movement and to minimise the danger of limbs flailing. In 1955 the GQ Parachute Company introduced combined parachute and seat fastenings for the Folland ejector seat instead of the two separate harnesses. The trend has been in recent years for flying-clothing designers to integrate clothing and equipment, and this is an example of where one piece of equipment has taken the place of two, thus making life much easier and more comfortable for the pilot. In the Martin-Baker Seat Mk 4 installed in Jet Provosts and Lightnings, the two harnesses were also combined into one. The combined harness was attached to the seat by two locks in the rear of the seat pan and another lock at shoulder height, these locks as well as the leg restraints being released by a time-release unit at the correct moment after ejection. When the Phantom was introduced in Britain the American torso harness was adopted and was later used in the Harrier, Buccaneer and Jaguar. This harness is put on in the crewroom and connected to the seat and parachute when strapping in, but because so many harnesses had to be issued (since there are more men than aircraft), and because their advantages did not outweigh those of the seat-mounted harnesses, the RAF is now reverting to the use of a simplified, combined, seat-mounted harness which will be installed in the Hawk, Phantom, Harrier, Buccaneer and Jaguar as well as in the Tornado.

The pilot and 'G' forces

One of the main physiological problems encountered on ejection is that of 'G'. The power of ejection has to be restricted within the limitations of the pilot's tolerance. Much valuable work was carried out by Martin-Baker using special rigs to determine tolerable 'G' forces. It was decided that a peak acceleration of 21'G' for one-tenth of a second should not be exceeded. From 15 to 20'G' is also experienced when the parachute opens. The force of the parachute's opening increases with altitude. High 'G' levels have to be of a very short duration if they are not to cause injury. A greater hazard is that of negative 'G' experienced with downward ejection. This form of escape was practised by the American Air Force with aircraft such as the Lockheed F104A and C Starfighter. However, a human frame can tolerate only small amounts of negative 'G', furthermore, the risks of ejecting at low level were greatly multiplied. Yet another version of assisted escape is the escape capsule used in the Bell X2, the B58 Hustler and the F111. This closed system of escape solves the problem of wind-blast at supersonic speeds and obviates the need for pressure suit, parachute or immersion suit since the capsule can build up its own pressure. But the many seeming advantages barely outweigh the disadvantages; notably the vast cost, weight, the complexity of the system which is prone to error and the very high deceleration loads which are imposed on the crew.

The 'G' forces experienced on ejection, although high, are of a short-term nature. But the 'G' loads imposed during many standard manoeuvres in modern high-performance aircraft would cause the pilot to black out or become unconscious if he were not protected.

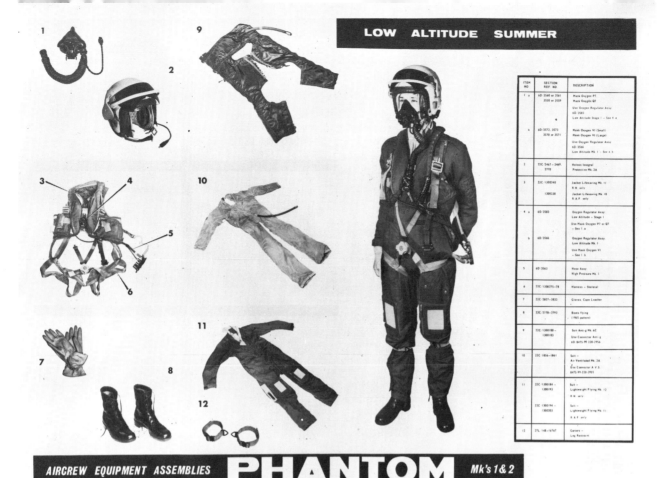

AIRCREW EQUIPMENT ASSEMBLIES **PHANTOM** Mk's 1 & 2

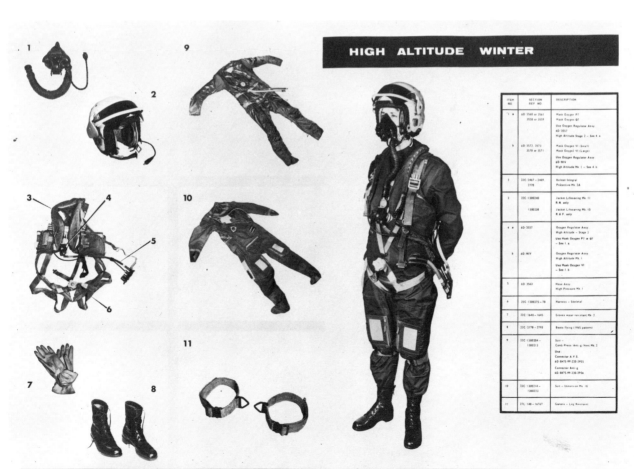

AIRCREW EQUIPMENT ASSEMBLIES **PHANTOM** Mk's 1 & 2

Some modern combat aircraft are stressed to an ultimate limit of 11 'G' whereas most pilots, even when wearing anti-'G' trousers, would black out within a matter of seconds when pulling 7'G' and would become unconscious at 8'G'. The pilot is restricted more by his physiological limitations than by the structural limitations of the aircraft.

The stronger airframes of the inter-war period had enabled aircraft to withstand stresses that could not be borne by the pilot. Germany pioneered research into the effects of 'G' on the human body and proposed that the pilot be enclosed in a water-filled suit. Research in Britain was on much the same lines, and in 1941 Squadron Leader W. R. Franks of the Royal Canadian Air Force introduced a water-filled anti-'G' suit. This was most cumbersome and proved just as effective when filled with air. From 1943 the University of Southern California began to make extensive studies into the effects of acceleration on the human body. They constructed a large human centrifuge and came up with the idea of using inflatable bladders and capstans to stem the flow of blood into the legs. This design principle was later incorporated in the American capstan partial-pressure suit. Anti-'G' suits were officially issued for use in active service by the Americans during the Korean War of 1950–3. Extending from the waist downwards the anti-'G' suit consisted of an abdominal bladder and capstans which inflated automatically from the engine's compressor system whenever the acceleration exceeded 2'G'. This restriction prevented the blood from pooling in the lower half of the body and so raised the wearer's resistance to black-out and reduced fatigue caused by repeated applications of 'G'. The F86 Sabre pilots found the suit unpleasant to wear since it imposed one lb per sq in of pressure for each 'G', but it undoubtedly saved many lives and meant that greater use could be made of the Sabre's performance capabilities.

American Navy pilots from the immediate post-war years.

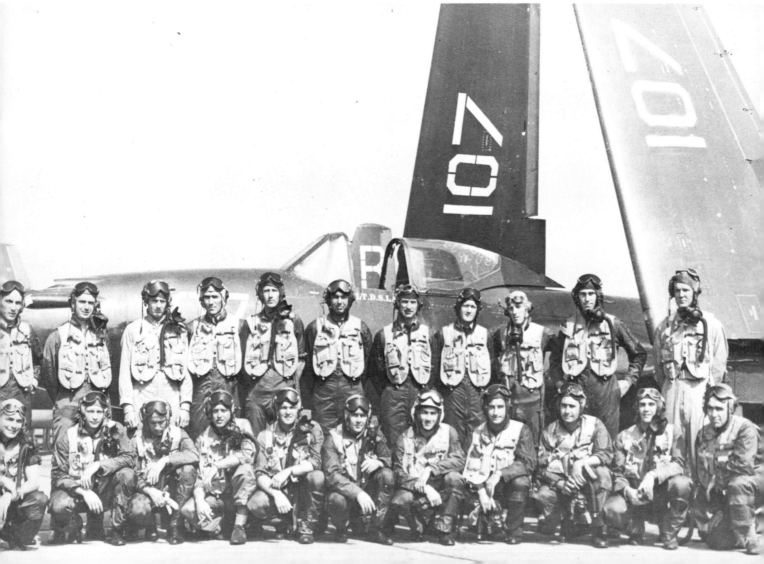

Anti-'G' trousers were introduced in the RAF in the early fifties; Javelin pilots were some of the first to be issued with them. The trousers were constructed of non-stretch nylon and fitted with sets of rubber air bladders over the abdomen, the outside of the thighs and the inside of the calves. The bladders inflated automatically whenever the force acting on the pilot exceeded 2'G', thus pulling the fabric of the trousers tight, which, in turn, applied pressure rather like the inflatable arm bandage used by a doctor when testing blood pressure. Anti-'G' trousers were always worn as part of the pressure-clothing assembly with the pressure waistcoat or jerkin for high-altitude flights. The Mks 6 and 7 anti-'G' trousers are used by pilots of modern military aircraft obliged to fly low if they intend to dodge radar. The anti-'G' partial-pressure and air-ventilated suits have since 1967 been combined into one piece of equipment for high-altitude opera-tions, and were initially used in the Phantom. While research has been continuing with the aim of increasing the comfort of the anti-'G' trousers (including the use of external anti-'G' trousers in hot climates), other experiments have been carried out in the attempt to find alternative solutions to 'G', including the prone and supine flying positions. A prone-pilot Meteor certainly raised the pilot's threshold to 'G' but the disadvantages of flying on one's tummy did not justify the adoption of this method.

High 'G' forces are imposed on naval aircrews when aircraft are catapulted off ships, however, these loads are imposed only for a matter of seconds and are therefore not critical. It has been proved that the effects of 'G' are mitigated by a correct and tightly fitting harness. This is certainly the case in the event of a crash, when high deceleration forces can be withstood by the pilot as long as he is firmly in his seat. So often a pilot withstands the great forces of a crash but is crushed by the instrument panel or seat.

Although the human body is unable to withstand as much negative 'G' as positive, it has rarely been the subject of lengthy research since most manoeuvres that produce negative 'G' such as outside loops, impose great stresses on both aircraft and pilot and are therefore infrequently performed. In recent years, however, much more attention has been focused on this aspect of 'G', since pilots of interceptor aircraft who abruptly change from a steep climb to level flight are subjected to this force. A negative-'G' strap helps to keep the pilot down in his seat. Negative 'G' causes the blood to concentrate in the head which results in an extremely unpleasant phenomenon known as 'red-out'. How-ever, this rise in blood pressure in the head is counteracted by the effects of a partial-pressure helmet which is worn on all high-altitude flights. Although many modern aircraft can withstand 'G' forces considerably in excess of those that the pilot can tolerate, pro-tective clothing and a sound understanding of his physiological limitations ensure man's mastery over his machine; the incorporation of a 'G' meter in the instrument panel acts as an added safeguard.

Although speed in itself in straight and level flight does not impose any physiological stress on the pilot it does tax his powers of concentration and reaction more than ever before. One may wonder why, since in modern times the pilot is greatly assisted by ground control as well as by the many dials on his instrument panel. However, the dials are extremely complex and demand his full attention and the faster he is travelling the quicker he must be able to react. Machines can now hurtle through the air at several times the speed of sound but man's powers of concentration and his reflexes are much the same as when he first took to the air in a balloon. A pilot of a high-performance aircraft must not only be able to react immediately to instructions from Air Traffic Control and to readings from his instruments, but he must also be permanently scanning the skies for other aircraft. There is an inevitable human time-lag between seeing a dot in the sky, recognising what it is and in what direction it is travelling, and taking avoiding action; but at high speeds this time-lag must be cut down to an absolute minimum. The eye also has to adapt rapidly from scanning the far distance of the sky to reading the instrument panel. This adjustment can take several seconds although the new 'head-up' display unit incorporated above the instrument panel of some military aircraft now means that the pilot does not have to look down to see essential information. The eye must also be able to adjust to different intensities of light. The glare reflected off clouds may be quite blinding, yet at great altitudes the sky may be a very dark blue, increasing the difficulty of seeing other aircraft. The limitations of the human eye were realised in the first all-jet aerial battles, in Korea. Here Mig 15s and F86 Sabres duelled in the skies at great speeds and altitudes, and within seconds of having searched a section of the sky a pilot could be under attack from an enemy aircraft which would seem to have appeared from nowhere.

Goggles were the standard form of eye protection until the early fifties, when visors were introduced. The Mk 1 visor was attached like goggles with an elasticised strap on to a helmet or bone-dome. Future Marks of visor would become integral with the bone-dome. Visors proved much more efficient than goggles since they provided a better field of vision and were easily adjustable to intermediate positions. The Mk 4 protective helmet in use today has one visor tinted against glare and an inner one made of poly-carbonate which serves to protect against ejection blast and bird-strike debris. It is worn normally in the down position throughout the flight. Recent advances in helmet accessories include the Marconi-Elliott helmet-mounted sight system. This complements the head-up display which gives information to the pilot while he is looking ahead. The sight system can give the pilot information warning him of any threat regardless of where he is looking and also enables him to designate targets to his avionic weapon-aiming system simply by looking at the target.

The Marconi-Elliott Helmet-Mounted sight system, which operates in conjunction with the Head Up Display.

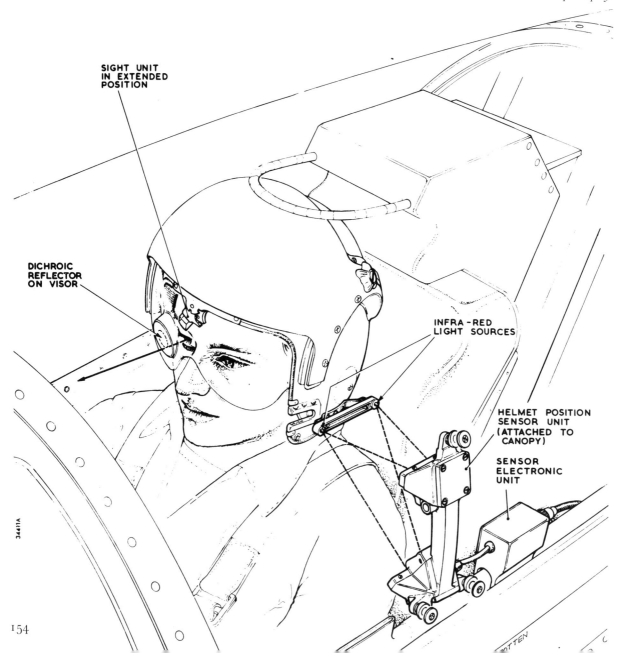

SIGHT UNIT IN EXTENDED POSITION

DICHROIC REFLECTOR ON VISOR

INFRA-RED LIGHT SOURCES

HELMET POSITION SENSOR UNIT (ATTACHED TO CANOPY)

SENSOR ELECTRONIC UNIT

34411A

The effects and treatment of heat

High-speed flight produces kinetic heating from skin friction; the faster an aircraft flies the hotter its skin temperature becomes. This is especially noticeable at lower altitudes. The heat penetrates the air-conditioned cockpit, but if the pilot is wearing many layers of protective clothing and the cockpit air conditioning is not working properly he will become extremely uncomfortable. For many reasons, for example heating from the avionics systems, the temperature of the cockpit can build up rapidly, especially when the aircraft is taxiing and waiting for take-off, to such an extent that the pilot can be in a state of virtual collapse. Thermal stress should be avoided at all costs since it reduces the pilot's powers of concentration and greatly impairs his reactions. It has been suggested that the heat to which a pilot is subjected when wearing an immersion suit can considerably reduce not only his concentration but also his tolerance to positive 'G'.

The RAF Institute of Aviation Medicine has done much research into the physiological effects of temperature extremes upon aircrews, and in the late 1940s came up with the idea of an air-ventilated suit for keeping the body cool and dry. This is a lightweight cotton or nylon suit, on the inside of which has been sewn a maze of small-diamter PVC tubes terminating in jets. The first suit was made for a speed-record flight over a desert in an early jet aircraft. It proved so successful that it was introduced into service. Air-ventilated suits are worn in many high-performance aircraft flying at low level, such as the Phantom and Buccaneer, in high- and medium-performance aircraft operating in tropical areas, under pressure suits in high-altitude aircraft, and very often under the sweaty immersion suits. When on stand-by, a ground trolley provides the necessary cooling. Once he is airborne the pilot is able to control the temperature of the air passing through the suit; warm air can be passed through the suit in the event of loss of cabin pressure at high altitude. The United States Air Force also has an air-ventilated suit but of a different design. Air flows *en masse* between two layers of impermeable material. The material is held apart by a form of corrugation incorporated into the material, and the air reaches the body through hundreds of minute holes in the inner lining. Air-ventilated suits, often known as 'fairy' suits, are not very popular because, unless portable conditioners are available for use in the crewroom and while checks are being carried out in the aircraft before take-off, the heat build-up caused by the suit can be so great that it tends to out-weigh any advantages of body-cooling once the wearer is airborne.

A different method of body-cooling was introduced in the mid sixties by Des Burton of Farnborough, who devised a liquid-conditioned suit in which liquid flows through a series of very small PVC pipes in closed circuit with an aircraft-mounted heat-exchanger. This method was successfully adopted by NASA for their Apollo space programme and is now being introduced into the RAF for use in the Tornado. The success of this suit lies in the fact that the heat-transfer properties of liquids are far superior to those of air.

Unlike in former days, modern pilots are subjected to uncomfortable excesses of heat more often than of cold. As a result, electrically heated clothing has been substantially phased out during the last decade. However, electrically heated socks and gloves are worn under immersion coveralls by airmen in Royal Naval helicopters. These crew members, and especially the winchman, can be subjected to extreme cold as they patrol the endless bitter wastes of the northern seas, often with the helicopter doors open.

The lot of the airman who flies for long periods over great expanses of sea has been further improved by the introduction of the immersion coverall popularly known as the 'goon' suit. Originally used by Hurricane pilots catapulted off merchant ships in the war, immersion coveralls protect the wearer from cold and exposure, both in the aircraft and after baling out or ditching, thus greatly increasing his expected survival time in cold water. The first post-war design, the Mk 7, was a two-piece suit which was unpopular since it took at least a quarter of an hour to put it on. The rubber extension of the jacket and trousers at the waist was meant to roll into a thin sausage but in fact appeared more like a large rubber tyre, and it was most uncomfortable for long periods of stand-by. A one-piece immersion coverall with attached water-proof socks has recently been introduced, the Mk 10, which is much more comfortable and easier to put on. Special water-proof and gas-tight zip-fasteners are used on all designs of immersion coverall. Both the Mk 7 and the Mk 10 coveralls are made of a ventile fabric which seals when in water to become wind- and water-proof and yet permits the fabric to breathe. They provide the necessary protection until the airman is able to get into his dinghy. The degree of protection depends to a large extent on what is worn under the immersion coverall. This is normally an inner coverall with an Acrilan pile lining known as a 'bunny suit', worn on top of 'long johns'. The helicopter winchman's immersion coverall is similar to the Mk 10 but of traffic yellow rather than an olive-drab colour.

One automatically associates the post-war years particularly with jet aircraft, but the now-common helicopter did not make its début on a widespread scale until the close of the last war. The advantages of helicopters in jungle warfare were soon realised, and aircraft such as the Whirlwind, Dragonfly and Bristol Sycamore played an important role in Malaya, Korea and Suez. Today they are associated with courageous feats of life-saving and mountain rescue in Britain and with the relief of flooded and famine-stricken lands overseas. Mention has already been made of the protective clothing worn by helicopter crews flying over the chill, dark North Sea. Immersion clothing is obviously not required for operations over land but a standard piece of equipment worn by chopper crews the world over is a helmet with good noise exclusion. Helicopters are noisy, vibrating creatures, and without effective ear protection crew fatigue would soon set in.

Innovations

Many new items of flying clothing have been introduced since the last war to protect aircrew from the hazards of high-altitude and high-speed flight and ejection, hazards that had rarely been encountered before the advent of jet-propelled aircraft. But many other items of clothing developed only gradually from former designs. In the early fifties a wide-mesh string vest was introduced which had originally been designed for the Commandoes during the war. This popular piece of clothing is extremely efficient in maintaining a comfortable body temperature in both hot and cold climates. Acrilan pile underwear is, however, used in Arctic conditions and by North Sea helicopter crews. Lightweight flying overalls have remained much the same in design since the mid forties. For many years they were made of gabardine but are now made either from a mixture

A Nimrod crew in olive drab overalls and lif[e] preservers. In flight they would wear [a] headset.

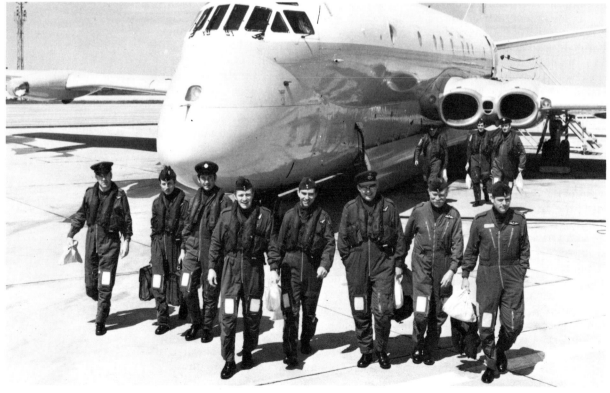

of flax and Terylene such as the RAF Mk II overall, or from a new material called Nomex which has fire-retardant properties and which, although more costly than flax/Terylene, is much more durable. Teklan is another material which resists ignition. However, these special materials provide protection for only a matter of seconds—the best method of fire protection is to wear as many layers of clothing as possible. Until the mid-sixties most RAF flying clothing was issued in a distinctive blue-grey colour, but in recent years the flying clothing of all three Services has been very similar, the more usual colour being an olive-drab or a jungle-green, although camouflage-pattern overalls are sometimes worn by aircrew. This is partly because all Service flying clothing is now issued from one source and partly because it has to conform with NATO requirements. Brevet 'wings', rank and squadron badges are always sewn onto the overalls.

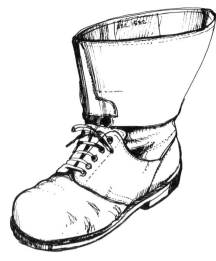

1952 Pattern Boot, made of polished black leather.

Ergonomics have played an important part in the design of modern flying overalls. Today's coveralls have nine pockets, each specially positioned and designed to accommodate maps, gloves, a first-aid kit, pen, pencil and torch as well as a writing pad. Writing pads, used to note down the controller's instructions, were originally pads of paper that could be attached onto the flying suit. But in the late fifties a Perspex window and China-graph were substituted. These windows are incorporated on the suit immediately above the wearer's knees. More attention has been paid to ensuring that there are no loose articles or flapping pieces of material. Even a loose pencil could be distracting, if not actually dangerous, in flight. Velcro provides a safe and easy method of closing pockets and securing loose straps. Buttons are rarely used, since a loose button can jam the controls. When buttons are used they are attached by tape rather than thread.

The late inter-war trend to integrate a parachute harness, life-jacket and flying suit has continued in the post-war period. These suits are used mainly by aircrews who have to move around inside the aircraft and do not want to be hampered by the weight and bulk of a parachute. In an emergency a chest-type pack is clipped on. As well as the normal pockets, provision is also made in the suit for escape and survival aids, including an emergency oxygen supply, a whistle, knife, search and rescue and homing equipment, a lamp, heliograph and fluorescine pack.

In 1951 a cold-weather flying suit was introduced for aircrews operating in arctic-like climates. This replaced the 1941-pattern flying suit and kapok-quilted lining as well as the Irvin suit. Although the Irvin suit had not been issued since 1943 many airmen continued to wear their old jackets throughout the later forties. The cold-weather flying suit consisted of a hip-length jacket made of blue-grey or olive-drab wind-proof gabardine lined with a woollen material and fitted with a hood. The gabardine trousers were also supposed to be wind-proof. However, the suit was unpopular because it was draughty and appeared to be no improvement on previous designs.

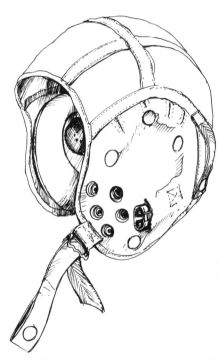

Type G helmet. Designed to be worn with the Mk 1 and Mk 1A Bone Dome, it is made of a grey/blue cotton cellular material, differing very slightly from the earlier Type F helmet. These helmets had large, comfortable ear pads which were glycerine filled, allowing them to take up the contours of the wearer's head. The Type G helmet was introduced in the early 1950's.

Gloves have changed little since wartime days, whereas flying boots have progressed from the 1943-pattern, black leather escape boot. The 1952-pattern boot was a more streamlined version of the 1943 boot. It had a full leg to allow the trousers to be tucked in, and the upper section of the boot could be removed to avoid embarrassment if you came down in enemy territory; but it was by no means ideal. Ian Weston, an ex-RAF pilot and former member of the Rothman's Aerobatic Team recalled wearing the 1952-pattern boots one winter in Germany. The uppers were so baggy that on walking out to the aircraft they filled with snow, which promptly melted, causing much discomfort. They were also renowned for coming off altogether in the event of a high-speed ejection. The 1965-pattern boot to some extent remedied these defects as it is tighter fitting than the 1952-pattern. With full lace-up closure, it stays on during ejection and also has a specially designed tread to avoid picking up pebbles, etc that may work loose during flight. A special lightweight flying boot has been introduced for wear in temperate summer conditions.

Leather flying helmets have been replaced by the multi-purpose, fibreglass bone-dome, although the G Type fabric helmet or a headset is used by many airmen in transport aircraft. Communication equipment has also improved significantly, eliminating external noises and making speech more audible, although the glycerine-filled earpads of more recent bone-domes are not averse to leaking. Goggles are still used to simulate certain conditions during flying training, such as night-vision training goggles or instrument-flying practice goggles.

Late developments

The post-war years have seen a much more scientific approach to flying clothing. Clothing is designed not simply to be functional but also to be comfortable. The significant work carried out in the field of aviation medicine, the development of man-made fibres and the progress in clothing technology have made these advances possible. Anthropometry or the precision sizing of clothing is a new word heard in connection with modern flying clothing. No longer are aircrews issued with kit straight off the shelf in a matter of minutes. Today's aircrews spend several days at the Aero Medical Training Centre at RAF North Luffenham, where they are measured from head to foot and precisely fitted with their exclusive and expensive wardrobe. The aircrews are also given a thorough medical examination and are lectured on all aspects of aviation medicine so that they can understand their bodies' reactions to flight and recognise dangerous physiological situations. There is an Aircrew Equipment Assembly list for each aircraft type, as the requirements, for example, of a VC10 navigator and a Jaguar pilot are very different.

A Sukhoi Su-7, probably in Syria, with aircrew dressed in Russian clothing.

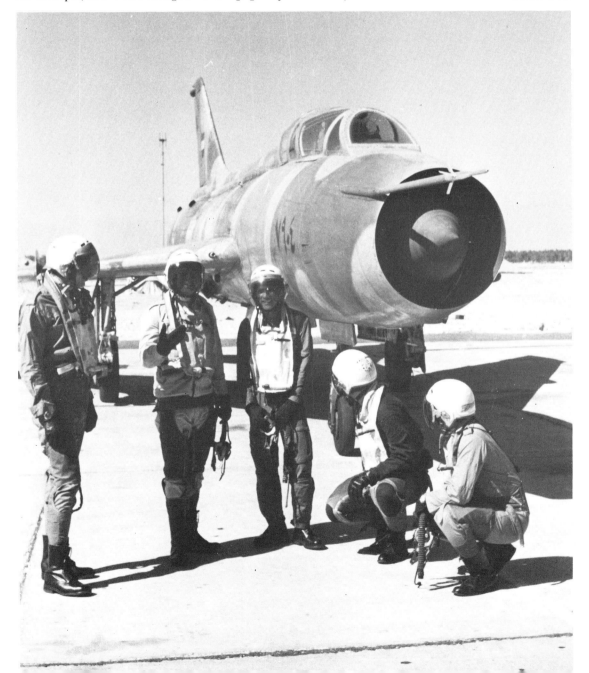

Private pilots are also becoming increasingly aware of safety requirements and of man's physiological limitations. Small oxygen supplies are carried in aircraft likely to fly over 10,000ft. This knowledge is especially pertinent in the case of record-breaking balloon and glider pilots who easily attain altitudes where oxygen is required and sometimes reach heights where pressure-breathing equipment is necessary. Weight restrictions may preclude the incorporation of cockpit heating equipment in these craft so the hazards of cold must be well appreciated and every precaution taken. Glider pilots wear as many layers of thin clothing as possible, often including a pair of tights. Pilots and passengers of light aircraft have no need to wear special flying clothing as such, although the wearing of any nylon clothing is inadvisable since it can cause extremely serious damage to the body in the event of a fire; nylon socks and watch straps are particularly vulnerable. The Civil Aviation Authority has also shown its awareness of safety requirements for private pilots for, as from January 1978, shoulder harnesses have to be installed at the pilots' seats of all British registered aircraft to provide upper torso restraint.

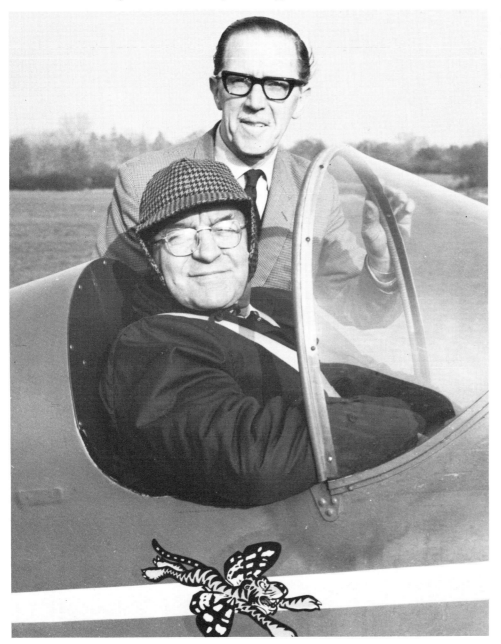

Norman Jones and Chris Wren. A deerstalker hat and anorak provide adequate protection against the cold encountered at the relatively low altitudes where the private pilot flies.

The private pilot, as well as the commercial pilot and his passengers, are much better off today than they were sixty years ago. They now have the protection of an enclosed cockpit and no longer have to bundle themselves up in layer upon layer of clothing, supplemented by hot-water bottles, and ear-bungs. The military pilot's clothing on the other hand has, of necessity become increasingly specialised and complex in line with the development of ever more sophisticated flying machines. There is no such thing as shirt-sleeve flying in a high-performance aircraft, nor can an officer go to war, as Sir Richard Atcherley once suggested 'dressed like a Christian gentleman'. Instead, specially designed and carefully fitted clothing serves to protect the airman against every conceivable emergency condition and keeps him alive in a hostile environment, sometimes to the detriment of his comfort, for the clothing can be restricting, and very often too warm. Much work is being done to increase aircrew comfort by improving the general design of the clothing and the materials used, for officialdom has gradually recognised that the efficiency of aircrews depends on their comfort in the air and arrangements for their survival in emergency. There are also new problems to be solved. For example it is realised that future conflicts may involve nuclear, biological or chemical warfare, and suitable protective clothing is being designed for wear in the air as well as on the ground. Aircrews, aviation doctors and flying-clothing designers do not always see eye to eye but on one point they would all agree, that there is still a future for flying clothing.

Appendix I

Stores Reference Numbers for Flying Clothing

This is a guide to RAF stores reference numbers applied to flying clothing officially issued to RAF aircrew up to 1965. All flying clothing has a 22C prefix. This list does not include oxygen equipment which has a 6D prefix or electrical head equipment which has a 10A prefix.

22C/1	Belts, life-saving, self inflating, Type A–Perrins
2	Boots, airship–(obs 1924)
3	Boots, flying, knee (obs 1924)
4	Boots, flying, thigh
5	Caps, fur-lined
6	Gauntlets, flying
7	Glasses non-tinted
8	Glasses, tinted
9	Gloves, silk
10	Goggles, mask, Mk I (obs 1924)
11	Goggles, mask Mk II
12	Helmets, aviation (obs 1924)
13	Helmets, flying, cork, aviation,–issued E of Malta for summer wear –Type A
14	Jackets, flying, leather–long (obs 1924)
15	Jacket, life saving–Anliffe pattern (obs 1924)
16	Belts, life-saving–Boddy (obs 1932)
17	Waistcoats, life-saving–Gieve, with flask
18	Jackets, life saving, heavy (obs 1932)
19	Jackets, life-saving–Read pattern (obs by 24)
20	Linings, worsted, gauntlet
21	Overshoes, gaitered
22	Suits, aviation, fireproofed, Sidcot
23	Sweaters, aviation (obs 1924)
24	Trousers, leather (obs 1924)
27	Case for glasses
29	Jackets, flying, leather, short (obs 1932)
30	Waistcoats, life-saving, inflatable–Belt pattern, Gieve (obs 1932)
31	Waistcoats, life-saving–Boddy pattern

45	Belt, life-saving, self-inflating Type B (obs. 1932)	
49	Boots, flying knee—1930-pattern	
50	Socks	
51	Cap, furlined—1930-pattern	
52	Collar, flying suit—1930-pattern	
53	Lining inner, flying suit—1930-pattern	
54	Suit outer, flying suit—1930-pattern	
55	Waistcoat, life-saving, inflatable—stole-pattern (intd 1932)	
57	Flaps for (51)	
58	Left-hand gauntlet	
59	Right-hand gauntlet	
60	Left-hand gauntlet—1933-pattern	
61	Right-hand gauntlet—1933-pattern	
62	Goggles—Mk IIIA (c. 1934)	
63	Windows for goggles—Mk IIIA	
64	Helmet, flying—Type B	
65	Helmet, flying	
66	Zip-ear unit for helmet	
67	Pad, rubber for, 22C/66	
68	Protector, face (to snap over press-studs), chamois	
69	Goggles Mask—Mk III—for high-altitude flying (Mk IICL*)	
70	Fasteners, oxygen-tube	
72	Stole for waistcoat, life-saving	
77	Snap-fasteners	
79	Waistcoat, life-saving—stole-pattern, tropical	
80	Boots, flying, knee—1936-pattern	
82	Windows, tinted, for (62) and (69)	
83		
84		
85		
90		
95		
98	Jacket for suits, flying, thermally insulated	For high-altitude
99	Trousers for suits, flying, thermally-insulated	flying where cock-pit heating is inadequate (c. 1938)
101	Spectacles—Mk Va	
111	Goggles—Mk IV	
163	Boots, flying, brown, heated	
167	Goggles—Mk IVb	
234–242	Socks, lambswool (insoles for boots), sizes 5–12	
243–250	Gloves, flying, electrically heated—12 volts	
251–258	Gloves, flying, electrically heated—24 volts	
259–263	Gloves, silk, sizes 8–10	

873–874	Holders, tinted, for 930
875	Goggles, dark adaption—Mk1A
876	Windows, filter red, for 875
877–880	Helmets, leather—Type C, sizes 1–4
882	Spectacles—Mk VI Polaroid
883	Spectacles—Mk VIa Crookes B2
917–924	Boots, flying—1943-pattern, sizes 5–12
930	Goggles—Mk VIII
932	Goggles, gunnery night simulation
933–940	Socks, for boots—1943-pattern
948	Knife, for boots—1943-pattern
961–962	Spectacles—Mk8
969–972	Helmets, cotton drill—Type D, sizes 1–4
973–976	Helmets, Airtex—Type E, sizes 1–4
982	Frame for 930 c/w elastic headband
986–991	Gloves, gauntlet, sizes 7½–10, same as 22C/767–772
992–993	Gloves, chamois leather, sizes 9½–10
994	Spectacles—Mk 9
995	Spectacles—Mk 9A
1003	Ventilator tube, for 22C/862
1040	Goggles, night-vision training—indoor, for 22C/862
1041	Goggles, night-vision training—outdoor, for 22C/862
1042	Goggles, night-vision training—general, for 22C/862
1043	Disc, anti-mistant
1089–1093	Filter windows for goggles, instrument flying practice—Mk I
1104	Filter, blue, complete, for 22C/1136
1106–1108	Filters, for 22C/1136
1106–1108	Filters, blue, for 1136
1121–1126	Gloves, cape, leather, lightweight, with gauntlet, size 7½–10
1136	Goggles, instruments, flying-practice, frame—Mk 2
1137–1144	Overalls, flying, lightweight—1951-pattern
1161	Braces for overalls, flying, cold-weather
1162–1164	Vests, string—1951-pattern (cold- and extreme cold-weather clothing)
1153–1160	Cold weather overall—Mk I
1161	Braces, for cold weather overall
1165–1174	Shirt, aircrew, (extreme cold-weather clothing)
1175–1178	Jerseys, pullover (extreme cold-weather clothing)
1179	Scarf, neck square (extreme cold-weather clothing)
1186	Whistle
1188–1195	Drawers, pyjama-type (cold- and extreme-weather clothing)
1196–1198	Wristlets, woollen—1951-pattern (cold- and extreme cold-weather clothing)
1233–1240	Parkas, outer (cold- and extreme cold-weather clothing)
1241–1246	Mukluks (cold- and extreme cold-weather clothing)

1247–1252	Socks, duffel (cold- and extreme cold-weather clothing)
1253–1258	Insoles for Mukluks
1259–1263	Socks, plain knit (inner two pairs)
1264–1268	Socks, ribbed knit (the outermost pair)
1269–1271	Mitts, inner, woollen (cold- and extreme cold-weather clothing)
1272–1274	Mitts, outer, leather (cold- and extreme cold-weather clothing)
1275–1285	Caps, cold-weather, sizes $6\frac{1}{2}$–$7\frac{3}{4}$
1286–1288	Gloves, working (cold- and extreme cold-weather clothing)
1349	Jacket, life-saving—Mk 3
1351	Visor, flying, light screen—Mk I (RAF)
1352	Visor, flying, light screen—Mk IA (RN)
1369–1370	Spectacles, anti-glare—Mk 11
1371–1374	Waistcoats, pressure—Mk 1A
1377	Spectacles—Mk 12
1378	Spectacles—Mk 12A
1385–1388	Helmets, flying—Type F
1389–1392	Helmets, fabric portion of Type F
1398	Spectacles, Type G, large and 22C/1398 medium
1400–1415	Boots, flying—1952-pattern, sizes 5M–12L
1475–1478	Drawers, cotton, short, (for wear with air-ventilated suit)
1480	Jacket, life-saving—Mk 4
1495–1501	Drawers, aircrew, cotton, long (for wear with pressure clothing)
1502–1508	Vests, cotton, aircrew (for wear with pressure clothing)
1509–1512	Suits, flying, anti-G—Mk 4A
1515–1526	Helmets, flying, protective—Mk 1A
1527–1542	Boots, flying, rubber-soled
1543–1544	Suits, exposure, inflatable—Mk 2
1545–1563	Suits, partial-pressure
1597–1606	Shirt, aircrew, cotton, collar-attached (for wear with partial-pressure suit)
1632–1639	Boots, rubber—Mk 3 (for immersion suit—Mk 7)
1640–1645	Gloves, cape, leather, water-resistant (for immersion suit—Mk 7)
1648–1651	Screens, anti-glare, dark and light, for visors—Mk 2
1655	Visor, flying, dark screen—Mk IB (RAF)
1656	Visor, flying, dark screen—Mk IC (RN)
1657–1666	Shirts, aircrew (cold- and extreme cold-weather clothing)
1667–1670	Jerseys, pullover—1954-pattern (cold- and extreme cold-weather clothing)
1681–1682	Mittens—Mk 3 (for immersion suit—Mk 7)
1683	Flying clothing holdall
1686–1693	Jackets, cold-weather—Mk 1
1694–1701	Trousers, cold-weather—Mk 1
1712	Scarf, blue-grey, for wear with suit, flying—Mk 2
1713–1724	Jerkins, pressure—Mk 1
1725–1728	Helmets, flying—Type G
1729–1732	Helmets, fabric portion of Type G

1733–1738	Air-ventilated suit—Mk 2
1801–1814	Suits, aircrew, flying dress—Mk 2, blouse
1815–1828	Suits, aircrew flying dress—Mk 2, trousers
1841–1844	Suits, flying, anti-G—Mk 5A
1856–1861	Air-ventilated suit—Mk 2A
1863	Jacket, life-saving, passenger
1873	Maps, clip
1875	Outfit, anti-mist, for 930
1877	Jacket, life-saving—Mk 4A
1904–1911	Suits, flying—Mk 2, blue-grey linen
1928–1942	Suits, aircrew, flying-dress—Mk 2A, blue-grey, blouse
1943–1957	Suits, aircrew, flying-dress—Mk 2A, blue-grey, trousers
1958–1965	Suits, flying—Mk 4, blue-grey, cotton gabardine
1996	Knife, emergency, aircrew—Mk 2
2001–2006	Suits, flying—Mk 5, c/w lining
2008–2014	Jerkins, pressure—Mk 3
2016–2022	Jerkins, pressure—Mk 3
2024	Garters, leg-restraining, with quick-release D ring
2073–2078	Linings for suit, flying—Mk 5
2079–2090	Helmets, flying, parachutist
2093–2105	Helmets, flying, partial-pressure—Type E
2110–2124	Helmets, flying, protective—Mk 1A, c/w track and mechanism
2206–2220	Suits, electrically heated
2236–2238	Vests, Acrilan pile, sleeved (for winchmen and navigators in SAR helicopters)
2239–2241	Drawers, long, Acrilan pile (for winchmen and navigators in SAR helicopters)
2244	Visor, instrument-flying practice—1961, Type B
2245–2256	Jerkins, pressure—Mk 4
2271	Respirator, aircrew, ani-gas
2272	Visor, instrument, flying-practice—Type A
2274	Jacket, life-saving—Mk 7
2296–2309	Helmets, flying, parachutist, Army-type
2323–2325	Helmets, flying, protective—Mk 2
2329–2336	Smock denison, airborne troop
2342	Jacket, life-saving, parachutist
2376–2381	Screens, visor, anti-blast, dark and light
2399–2401	Covers, visors, screen for helmets, protective—Mk 2 and 2A
2432–2433	Spectacles, anti-glare—Mk 14
2457–2460	Suits, flying, anti-G—Mk 4B
2461–2464	Suit, flying, anti-G—Mk 5B
2467–2469	Helmet, flying, protective—Mk 2A
2486–2489	Suits, flying, immersion, helicopter—Mk 1
2491–2499	Overalls, parachute, jumping instructors

Appendix II

Notes on the conservation of flying clothing

Clothing should not be subjected to damp conditions, excessive heat or to bright light. It should be stored in a stable environment rather than in a room which is sometimes cold and damp and at other times very warm. Good ventilation and not too high a relative humidity prevents the growth of mould and bacteria. It is, therefore, inadvisable to seal clothing in airtight polythene bags, where condensation can occur.

As far as possible the clothing should be clean, for dirt encourages moths. It is preferable to have the work done by a specialist dry-cleaner rather than to attempt to clean or wash the garments yourself. They should then be hung on a coat-hanger and covered with a polythene bag to protect them from dirt. There should be a few air holes punched in the bag for ventilation and some para-dichlorobenzene crystals (moth-balls) put in the bottom of the bag or hung from the coat-hanger.

Leather coats, jackets and helmets have to be treated with care as they can easily dry out, harden and crack. Once the leather has lost its fibrous structure it is impossible to put new life into it, but if the leather is just rather hard, its flexibility can be restored by applying leather dressing. A preparation called *Pliantine* is ideal and can be obtained from

> Arthur Rich and Partners Limited
> 42 Mount Pleasant Drive
> Belper
> Derbyshire

This should be applied very sparingly and rubbed well in. Neatsfoot oil or saddle soap would also serve the same purpose.

Much of leather used for flying clothing is known as chrome leather. This means that it has been mineral-tanned rather than vegetable-tanned. The skin is treated with a salt of chromium to make it impervious to water while remaining pliable. Chrome leather is virtually non-wettable and is very durable, resisting attack by moulds and pollutants in the air. Leather coats are less likely to harden and crack if kept on a coat-hanger rather than folded away in a drawer. They should never be stored in very warm conditions.

Rubber items such as oxygen masks are the biggest problem, as once rubber has started to deteriorate it is impossible to inhibit. Ideally they should be kept in stable conditions and away from the light.

Appendix III

Loss of consciousness within several seconds.   **40,000** / **12 000**

Loss of consciousness after one minute.   **35,000** / **10 500**

Convulsions - loss of consciousness after a few minutes.   **30,000** / **9 000**

Unco-ordinated movements - emotional fits - loss of muscular control.   **24,500** / **7 500**

Weakened memory - false sensation of happiness - reduced concentration.   **20,000** / **6 000**

Impaired judgement - fatigue - headache.   **15,000** / **4 500**

13,000 / **4 000**

Fatigue after several hours.   **10,000** / **3 000**

Reduced night vision.   **5,000** / **1 500**

0

feet
metres

Oxygen–diagram of critical heights and their effects on the human consciousness.

168

Bibliography

There is a significant gap in existing literature where flying clothing is concerned. To complete the text for this book the authors have read countless biographies and auto biographies on the subject of flying and were able to piece together from odd sentences, a feel for the environment and some of the personal problems associated with flying clothing. More authoritative works on aerial warfare provided the necessary historical data, but it was only by reference to the incomplete records surviving in the Public Records Office, Ministry of Defence departments and document collections such as that of the Royal Air Force Museum, that any form of chronological sense could be produced.

A small bibliography is presented but this in no way reflects the great number of volumes used in some small way for our researches.

Winged Victory, V. M. Yeates, Cape, London, 1961.
Ginger Lacey—Fighter Pilot, R. Townshend Bickers, Hale, London, 1962.
The Royal Flying Corps, Sir R. Thompson, Leo Cooper, London, 1968.
Flying the Arctic, G. H. Wilkins, G. P. Putams' Sons, New York, 1928.
British Test Pilots, G. Dorman, Forbes Robertson, London, 1950.
Richthofen, W. R. Burrows, Hart-Davis, London, 1970.
Fringe of the Clouds, Sir P. C. Livingstone, Johnson, London, 1962.
The Dangerous Skies, A. E. Clouston, Cassell, London, 1954.
Enemy Coast Ahead, Guy Gibson V.C., Michael Joseph, London, 1946.
Luftwaffe Air Crews—Battle of Britain, B. L. Davis, Arms & Armour, London, 1974.
Aeromedicine for Aviators, K. E. E. Read, Airlife.
Medical Aspects of Aviation, E. Jokl, Pitman, 1943.
Doctors in the Air, Wing Commander R. Maycock, A.F.C., George Allen and Unwin, 1957.

Acknowledgements

There are many people who, over the years that we have been working on this book, have greatly helped and encouraged us. People who have worn flying clothing as well as those who have designed, tested and manufactured it have spent precious hours recounting the pros and cons of different items of clothing. Some have helped us with photographs, with identification of clothing or checking of text, others explaining technicalities of the clothing or even squeezing us into it and kindly letting us try it out for ourselves. The staff at the R.A.F. Museum at Hendon have been particularly helpful and our families extremely forebearing. We would like to thank all these people, many of whose names appear below, and most especially Mrs. Linda Howes for deciphering our handwriting and typing the text.

Group Captain M. K. Adams, AFC. Aircraft and Armament Experimental Establishment, Boscombe Down. Australian Archives. Australian War Memorial, Canberra. Aviation Medicine Training Centre, R.A.F. North Luffenham. Beaufort Air-Sea Equipment Ltd. John Blake. Boeing Commercial Airplane Co. British Aircraft Corporation Ltd. British Airways. John W. Brooks. J. M. Brooks. Burberrys Ltd. Canadian War Museum. Central Flying School. L. R. Dixon. Dunlop Ltd. Flight International. Wing Commander A. Golding-Barrett. Dr. Helen Grimshaw. Mrs E. Hannaford. R. C. Harrall. Hawker Siddeley Aviation Ltd. Helmets Ltd., Wheathamstead. Her Majesty's Stationery Office. Imperial War Museum. Irvin Great Britain Ltd. F. E. Lamplaugh. J. Lawrance. Lockheed Corporation. R. C. London. Major C. W. A. Lyons. M. L. Avistion Ltd. McDonnell Douglas Corporation. Marconi-Elliott Avionic Systems Ltd., Rochester. Martin-Baker Aircraft Co. Ltd. Fred May. The late Captain G. F. Meager A.F.C. Mine Safety Appliances Co. Ltd. Ministry of Defence. M.O.D. Procurement Executive RDAE1 and EP2. Wing Commander M. Morris, A.F.C. The Museum of the Corps of Royal Engineers. National Air and Space Museum, Washington. National Museum of Science and Technology, Canada. Count O'Brien of Thomond. Edgar Percival. Graham Potts. Alfred Price. Public Record Office. T. Quin-Hall. Radio Times Hulton Picture Library. Dr K. E. E. Read. E. A. Rokicki. Royal Aero Club. Royal Aeronautical Society. R.A.F. Central Flying School. R.A.F. Institute of Aviation Medicine. R.A.F. Museum, Hendon. Royal Aircraft Establishment, Farnborough. Royal Australian Air Force Museum, Point Cook. The Science Museum, London. The Science Museum of Victoria, Australia. Shelia Scott. Scott Polar Research Institute. Air Vice Marshal J. de M. Severne, MVO,OBE,AFC. Wing Commander R. R. Stanford-Tuck, DSO,DFC. Triplex Safety Glass Co. Ltd. United States Navy. Wing Commander Unwin. Lord Ventry. L. Walters. Ian Weston. Air Marshal Sir Richard Williams, KBE. The late Captain T. B. Williams, AFC. The Wright-Patterson Air Force Museum.

The extract from "Rocket Fighter" by Mano Ziegler, published by Macdonald and Jane's Publishers Ltd.

The extract from "Aviator Extraordinary" by Ralph Barker, published by Chatto and Windus Ltd.

Photographic Acknowledgements

The authors wish to acknowledge with thanks the following who have supplied the photographic material for "Flying Clothing".

Boeing Commercial Airplane Company: 138, 142.

Lord Braybrooke: 27.

British Aircraft Corporation: 77.

British Airways: 63, 133, 134, 135.

Mr J. M. Bruce: 16, 47, 70.

Burberrys Limited: 6, 24, 25, 31

F. E. Dymond: 92 *right*.

Flight International: 15, 19 *top*, 53 *right*, 105 *bottom*, 116, 158.

Imperial War Museum: 34, 35, 36, 37, 40, 42 *right*, 43, 45, 84, 85, 86, 88, 89, 90, 92 *left*, 93, 94, 100 *right*, 104, 105 *top*, 106, 108 *right*, 109, 110, 111, 115.

Lockheed Corporation: *Chapter 6 introduction photograph*, 67, 139, 141.

Marconi-Elliott Avionic Systems Limited: 154.

Martin Baker Engineering: 145, 147.

MacDonnell Douglas Corporation: 152.

K. M. Molson: 33 *bottom*.

Alfred Price: 98.

Punch Magazine: 39.

Group Captain W. S. O. Randle.

Radio Times Hulton Picture Library: 4, 5, 7, 10 *left*, 18, 52, 53 *left*, 54, 55 *bottom*, 72, 73.

Royal Aero Club: *Chapter 1 introduction photograph*, 8 *left*, 9, 10 *right*, 12, 17, 19 *bottom*, 20, 46, 55 *top*, 69, 71, 75, 144, 159.

Royal Engineers Museum: 3.

R.A.F. Museum – Crown Copyright: 8 *right*, 25 *left*, 26, 27 *right*, 28, 29, 30, 32, 33 *top*, 48, 56, 57, 61, 65, 91, 96, 100 *left*, 107 *bottom*, 108 *left*, 125 *top*, *Chapter 5 introduction photograph*, 136, 137, 143, 146, 148, 151, 156.

Science Museum: 2.

Smithsonian Institution: 11, 13, 14, 41, 42 *left*, 59, 60, 62, 78, 87, 121, 123, 125, 126, 127, 140.

Triplex: 75.

Neill Bruce Photographic: 48, 57, 61.

M.L. Aviation: 146.

Index

Numbers in **bold** type refer to illustrations